医护英语水平考试办公室
医护英语水平考试教研中心　组织编写

METS
测试与评析

（一级）

Level 1

主　编　顾　萍　朱　兰
（以下排名以姓氏笔画为序）

副主编　王力维　刘春妹　罗海鹏
编　者　朱建芳　刘晓慧　刘　艳
　　　　李新利　陈丹丹　岳蕴之
　　　　赵　轶　唐小敏　蒋姗姗

南京大学出版社

图书在版编目（CIP）数据

METS 测试与评析. 一级 / 顾萍，朱兰主编. — 南京：
南京大学出版社，2018.4(2024.3 重印)
 ISBN 978 - 7 - 305 - 20022 - 9

 Ⅰ. ①M… Ⅱ. ①顾… ②朱… Ⅲ. ①医学－英语－水
平考试－自学参考资料 Ⅳ. ①R

 中国版本图书馆 CIP 数据核字(2018)第 062879 号

出版发行　南京大学出版社
社　　址　南京市汉口路 22 号　　　　　邮　编　210093
书　　名　**METS 测试与评析（一级）**
　　　　　METS CESHI YU PINGXI(YI JI)
主　　编　顾　萍　朱　兰
责任编辑　裴维维　　　　　　　编辑热线　025 - 83592123
照　　排　南京南琳图文制作有限公司
印　　刷　南京百花彩色印刷广告制作有限责任公司
开　　本　787×1092　1/16　印张 8.75　字数 224 千
版　　次　2018 年 4 月第 1 版　2024 年 3 月第 2 次印刷
ISBN 978 - 7 - 305 - 20022 - 9
定　　价　27.00 元

网址：http://www.njupco.com
官方微博：http://weibo.com/njupco
官方微信号：njupress
销售咨询热线：(025) 83594756

前　言

　　《METS测试与评析》1—4级系列丛书由医护英语水平考试办公室和医护英语水平考试教研中心组织编写,全国近20所各类医学院校50余名教师和专家参加编写和审稿工作。丛书对各级别 METS考试的特点分别进行综述,其中的相关试题严格按照2017年最新版《全国医护英语水平考试考试大纲》的要求进行设计,辅以较为详尽的分析和说明,并提供参考答案和作文范文,旨在帮助学生有效备考,顺利通过医护英语水平考试各级别的考试。本系列丛书既可供学生自主学习使用,又可以用作 METS 考试强化教材,也是英语教师开展METS考试研究的重要参考资料。

　　参加编写《METS测试与评析(一级)》的教师包括:主编:顾萍(南京医科大学)、朱兰(南京卫生高等职业技术学校);副主编:王力维(常州卫生高等职业技术学校)、刘春妹(江苏医药职业学院)、罗海鹏(江苏省南通卫生高等职业技术学校);编者:朱建芳(南京医科大学)、刘晓慧(南京卫生高等职业技术学校)、刘艳(南京卫生高等职业技术学校)、李新利(江苏医药职业学院)、陈丹丹(南京医科大学康达学院)、赵轶(秦皇岛市卫生学校)、岳蕴之(常州卫生高等职业技术学校)、唐小敏(江苏省南通卫生高等职业技术学校)、蒋姗姗(秦皇岛市卫生学校)。

目 录

医护英语水平考试一级考试综述

根据 2017 版医护英语考试（METS）新大纲要求，METS 一级考试（笔试）由听力（Listening）、阅读与写作（Reading and Writing）两部分构成。考试时间为 120 分钟，满分为 100 分。试卷结构，包括题型、题量、赋分、权重、考试时间等如下表所示：

		测试任务类型	为考生提供的信息	题目数量	原始分数	权重（%）	考试时间（分钟）
Ⅰ. 听力	Part One	信息匹配	单句或短对话	5	5	30	20
	Part Two	信息判断	长对话	5	5		
	Part Three	多项选择	独白或长对话	5	5		
	Part Four	填写表格	长对话	5	5		
Ⅱ. 阅读与写作	Part One	信息匹配	单词、短语与单句	5	5	55	70
	Part Two	信息匹配	单句与告示	5	5		
	Part Three	补全对话	长对话与单句	5	5		
	Part Four	信息判断	短文	10	10		
	Part Five	填词补文	短文	10	10		
	Part Six	短文写作	表格、便条、关键语句等	1	15	15	30
总计				55＋1	70	100	120

为了帮助考生复习应考，我们将试卷的两部分简述如下，内容包括考试要求、题型分析、真题简评、应试技巧介绍等。

一、听力（Listening）

根据新大纲要求，听力测试由 4 个部分组成，每部分 5 题，共 20 题，主要考查考生理解口头信息的能力。本部分考试时间为 20 分钟，分数权重为 30%。

Part One　信息匹配

第一部分为 5 个单句或 5 段医患或护患之间的简单对话（约 120 词），要求考生根据听到的信息辨识对话中"疼痛部位"等信息,并将这些信息与5位患者的名字相匹配。在给出的8个选项中,1个为示例答案,另有2个为干扰项。每段对话之间有3秒钟的间隔供考生答题。录音播放两遍。

从近几年的全真题来看,开篇的5段对话均较容易,内容为医生或护士询问患者症状的问题,患者描述自己的疼痛部位或病症部位,对话由一男一女进行一问一答;在回答中涉及疼痛或症状的部位均为身体部位,如 head, eye, ear, throat, mouth, tooth, neck, shoulder, arm, elbow, wrist, chest, ribs, stomach, abdomen, belly, waist, hip, back, leg, knee, ankle, foot, toe, joint 等。

因此,考生只要掌握基本的表达身体疼痛部位的医学词汇即能解题。首先,考生要充分利用播放指示语的时间迅速扫视8个身体部位名词;其次,要正确进行患者名字与疼痛部位之间的匹配,关键是要听懂患者对疼痛部位的表述。如果听不到疼痛部位名词,则需要考生根据症状的描述对患病部位进行推测,如听到 feel nausea and vomit,考生要理解这个症状表达的含义为"感到恶心并呕吐",故推测胃部(stomach)不适。这类考题难度较大,在一级考试中占比很少。

Part Two　信息判断

本部分要求考生根据听到的一段医患或护患之间的长对话(约150词),对相关事实性信息做出正误(True or False)判断。这段录音播放两遍,每遍播完后有10秒钟的间隔供考生答题。

信息判断题对话稍长,难度较第一部分有所增加。该部分听力主题以日常保健、医疗检查和常见疾病为主,一般都为与医学有关的常识性对话,不需要深奥的医学专业知识,但内容广泛,近几年真题主题涉及 a sleeping problem, high blood pressure, complaint of a cough, inpatient care, type one diabetes, injures related to falling down 等。考题设计以对事实或细节的正误判断为主,如:"The medicine should be taken twice a day." "The patient doesn't smoke now." "He has no breathing problem." 等;鲜有推理题或归纳题。可见,考题设计的难度并不大,建议考生利用播放指导语的时间阅读题干,画出关键词,根据题意,在听力中抓取对话的细节。

Part Three　多项选择

本部分要求考生根据听到的一段独白或长对话(约150词),辨识重要或特定的细节内容,并从所提供的3个选项中选择一个最佳答案。录音播放两遍,每遍播完有10秒钟的间隔供考生答题。

Part Three 和 Part Two 有相似之处,亦有诸多不同。相似之处在于,独白或长对话的长度类似,均为150词左右,考题均以事实题、细节题为主;而不同之处在于 Part Two 为正误判断题(True or False),而 Part Three 则为多项选择题。显然,Part Three 要难于 Part Two。此部分涉及的主题与第二部分类似,有常见疾病症状描述、医院常规检查、健康知识宣教和疾病预防等。从近年真题来看,主要考查了描述疼痛、医疗检查(如 MRI 核磁共振、CT 等)、出院后保健、成年人粉刺预防、头痛的治疗等。如前所述,Part Three 的考题多为事实题、细节题,如:"When does she have the pain?" "How severe is the pain?" "Which of the following is NOT the advice?"等。解答此类选择题,要求考生能够熟悉主题,对题干要求捕捉的信息提前预测,以便有所侧重地听,解题关键在于关注考题的关键信息,尤其是疾病名称、症状、疼痛部位、患病时长、用药信息等。

Part Four   填写表格

本部分要求考生根据听到的一段医患或护患之间的长对话(约 180 词),辨识重要或特定的信息,并根据听到的信息填写表格。这段录音播放两遍,每遍播完有 10 秒的停顿时间供考生答题。

表格填空题主要包括这几类:患者预约就医表、入院或出院信息登记表、患者检查记录表、生命体征监测表、转诊记录表等。从近几年的真题来看,考查了 admission card, appointment record, patient record 和 referral 等。这部分要求考生根据所听到的信息填写表格中空缺的 5 个词或短语,如姓名、性别、出生年月、体重、体温、脉搏、呼吸、血压、血氧饱和度、主治医生姓名、联系方式、亲属联系方式、就诊时间、随访时间等。一般而言,这些空缺的词或短语多数较为简单,姓名一般会重复一次或拼写,其他空格信息有日期的书写、身体疼痛部位、疾病症状、用药量、过敏食物或药物名称等,如:Williams, Nov. 22, milk, stomachache 等,个别空格会出现医学专业词汇,如:vomit, checkup 等,但以日常词汇为主。与听力的前三部分相比,第四部分要求考生能正确拼写听到的词汇;而拼写无疑是考生的弱项,这是第四部分的难点所在。解答过程中,考生应提前迅速浏览考题,对表格的主题和需要填写的信息有所了解,进行预测,听力过程中就能比较准确地定位信息,填出相关词语。

学习建议:

一级听力试题共四个部分:信息匹配、信息判断、多项选择和填写表格。我们在前面对上述各部分的题型及解题技巧等做了简略说明。这里尚有几点要再次强调一下。

首先,要充分利用发考卷后,播放每部分答题指导语的一段时间,快速阅读 Part Two, Part Three, Part Four 的题干,尽量画出关键词或易混词,从而预测听力内容,为答题做好准备,提高答题准确率。Part Three 是多项选择题,考生不仅应迅速阅读本部分 5 个句子,还应浏览每题中的 3 个选项,并做出合理预测。Part Four 是填写表格,解题关键在于拼写词语,考生应在平时重视单词的读音和拼写,对于重要的医学词汇,如身体部位、疾病名称、症状词汇要学习拼读,方能正确填出所听到的词或词组。

其次,在听录音时,最好能适当记录;用符号或首字母记下相关的数字、人名、地名、关键词、重要的细节等,勾出听到的选项,以便答题时有据可依。

最后,医学词汇的积累是提高听力能力的基础,要正确听读。错误或模棱两可的发音,会导致听力时无法辨认词义,造成错误。积累医学词汇时,一级考纲中涉及的身体部位、器官名称、疾病名称、医院科室、疾病症状等都是听力中的重点单词,要重点认读,以便在听力过程中快速地辨识出这些词汇的含义。

为了提高听力,考生平时应多看、多听英语节目,尝试听慢速 VOA 中的健康类节目、BBC 中的保健节目等,尤其是其中的健康类报道。只要持之以恒,坚持半年、一年,听力必有长进。

二、阅读与写作(Reading and Writing)

阅读与写作测试由 6 个部分组成,前 5 部分为阅读测试,第 6 部分为写作测试。阅读的 5 个部分主要考查考生理解书面信息的能力。这部分考试时间为 100 分钟,分数权重为 70%。

Part One 信息匹配

本部分考查考生辨识医学词汇的能力(约 50 词)。考生要将 5 个医学词汇的定义与 8 个选项中的正确单词或短语进行匹配,其中有 1 个示例的答案,还有 2 个干扰项。考查的医学词汇或短语有医疗器械、医疗场所、医疗操作等。

近几年的真题涉及的医学词汇和短语有 wheelchair, microscope, tablet, oxygen mask, forceps, ICU, IV bag, chart, operating room, monitor, ward, bedpan, ambulance, tweezers, ointment, probe, CT scan, syringe, walking frame, CPR, thermometer, injector, ultrasound 等,相应的表述如:"It is a device that fits over the nose and mouth to supply oxygen." 匹配"oxygen mask"。又如"It is a hard bandage that is wrapped around a broken bone to keep it in place." 匹配 "cast"。

这部分试题主要考查考生理解医疗器械、医学场所、医学操作表述的能力,从关键词中推测相应的医学名词或短语。因此,解题时要圈出 5 个题干中关键的名词或动词,以及理解 8 个选项的意思,这样才能正确匹配。建议考生对考纲中的医疗器械、医学场所、医学操作的词汇或词组进行整理,归类记忆,提高对于医学词汇的认知能力。

Part Two 信息匹配

本部分考查考生理解常见医学环境中简短信息(如告示、标识语、留言、广告、消息等约 80 词)的能力。题目要求考生将 5 句陈述与 7 条告示中的 5 条进行匹配,其中 1 个是示例的答案。

近几年来的真题涉及的标语或告示分为以下几类,如用药、保健、招聘医疗人员的网址、药品说明、药品保存指导、用药安全告示、饮食禁忌提示、保健建议、就医指导、治疗注意事项、医用垃圾告示、医疗场所说明、术前禁忌、医疗书籍概要、皮试指导、医疗仪器操作指导、探视时间、专科医院介绍等。相应的陈述如:"Avoid heavy exercise for 24 hours before exam." "External use only." 等。

这类信息匹配题要求考生理解选项中的标语含义,确认属于哪一类标语,是关于药品的还是关于保健禁忌的或是关于治疗护理指导等的,然后理解题干中的情境,部分简单的试题会在关键词上构成呼应,这可以作为匹配的线索,但最终确定选项要依靠整体理解。考生可以通过关注医院场所和药物上的英文标识提高辨识医学标识和告示的能力,经常积累这些标识中的短语词汇,积少成多,就能顺利解答此类题型。

Part Three 补全对话

本部分考查考生理解常见医学环境中会话文本(约 150 词)的能力。题目要求考生在阅读全文的基础上,根据上下文从 8 个选项中选出最佳答案,其中有 1 个是示例的答案,还有 2 个干扰项。

此部分类似于听力的第三部分,涉及的主题广泛,和医学保健有关的对话都有可能出现。因此考生可以参照考纲中"考试话题范围及交际任务"的条目,熟悉如医疗操作、问诊、主诉、常见疾病症状、术前指导、医疗检查注意事项、健康宣教等。对这些医学常识有所了解,答题时就能进行预测,提高正确率。

近几年来真题涉及以下主题,如保健宣教,饮食、运动禁忌,常见疾病(如感冒、咳嗽、胃疼、腹泻等)的问诊与检查,体检的注意事项,测量血压,心电图检查等。这部分的考题较为灵活,尤为体现考生的交际能力。考生要能够根据对话的上下文,推测需要选择的语句,在有干扰项的情况下,结合上文和下文的关键词,提炼对话精髓,不能答非所问。例如"—What seems to be bothering you? —I have had a bad cough for a few days."在答题过程中,如果发现有多个备选项符合上下文,可以考虑全篇对话,排除下文需要的选项。

Part Four　信息判断

本部分考查考生通过理解医学短文(约 200 词)获取重要信息的能力。要求考生在阅读全文的基础上,对给出的 10 个句子所表达的信息做出判断,有的信息是正确的,有的是错误的,有的文中没有提及。

阅读理解信息判断题型较常见,涉及的文章主题比较多,体裁多样,如对药品、疾病的说明文,医疗人员或患者描述性的记叙文,医学前沿动向的报道,对一个医学现象的论述文。一级考试着重基础,虽然主题和文体多样化,但考查的重点是考生理解与医疗健康有关常识性文章的能力,包括归纳全文大意、理解细节信息、推测作者意图等的能力。近几年的真题考查了这几个主题,如 children's dental health, the wonderful world of blood, the discovery of penicillin, how to stop nosebleed, punishment can worsen bedwetting, food and cancer 等。考题设计以细节信息题为主,如"Blood cells are red blood cells and white blood cells.",亦有推测题,如"Without platelets, blood can clot when we have a little cut."。

可见,考生首先要对医学领域的常识性知识(如常见疾病成因、治疗方式等)有所了解,具备了一定的背景知识能降低阅读的难度。其次,考生应该通读全文,把握文章的脉络和内在逻辑关系,具有较强的预测能力,能够结合上下文对细节信息准确的理解,根据题干或题干中的关键词锁定文中信息的出处,运用直接判断、排除、比较或逻辑推理推敲正误。正误判断题这种题型除 True, False 以外,还有 Not Given 这一选项。如果考生能够准确定位题干的信息在文中的出处,比较容易判断一个句子"正确"或"错误";但判断一个句子是否为"未提及"则比较困难。一般说来,所谓"错",一定是针对文中某个正确的陈述的错误,考生可以根据文章表述对"错误"选项进行更正;而"未提及"则与文章没有任何联系,不能由文章某些信息判断正确或错误。这就要求我们加强训练,提高对"错误"和"未提及"区别的敏感度。

Part Five 填词补文

本部分通过填充词汇考查考生理解文章（约 150 词）的能力。要求考生根据上下文从所给的 12 个选项中选择一个正确的词汇填入相应空白处，其中有 2 个为干扰项。

这类文章通常为介绍某位患者的病历或某种疾病的描述，主题具有明显的医学特征，空白处考查考生联系上下文理解医学信息的能力，文章结构严谨，层次分明，逻辑性强，能较好地检测考生把握文章总体结构及上下文逻辑关系的能力。近几年的真题均为医学短文，如病人病历、疼痛的症状、检查和治疗，情绪低落症状，甲状腺肿症状，慢性疼痛，儿童肥胖等，语言难度适中。

所谓填词补文，亦即完形填空。这种题型早已成为各类英语考试的重要题型。它强调考生对整体语篇的把握，着重考查考生综合运用语言知识的能力，包括语法结构分析能力、词语辨析能力、语篇理解能力、逻辑推理能力等；是一种有一定难度的障碍性阅读理解题。12 个单词难易搭配，一部分为医学词汇，一部分为表达医学意思的常用词汇，词性涉及广，包含名词、动词、形容词、副词、介词等。一般以考查基础医学词汇为主，如：disease, admit, suffer from, painful, hospitalize 等；有时会出现稍难一些的单词，如 inflammation, diagnose, incision 等，但所占比例较小，约十之一二。

填词补文是全卷中考查考生综合能力的一个题型，也是难点所在。考生要通读全文，弄清文章的大意，然后根据文章的主旨和发展脉络，逐一答题。另一种方法是不看全文，仅看首句和第一、二空便开始逐一答题。两种方法各有利弊，主要看个人习惯。无论采用哪种方法，重要的是理解全文，尤其是根据空白处的上下文预测该空白应填词语的词性和语法形式，以缩小选择范围。这是做填词补文的重要技巧之一。此外，答题时还要注意文章与题目、题目与题目间的照应关系，要前后参照，上下贯通，选择符合上下文的选项。

Part Six 写作

本部分考查考生书面表达的能力，要求考生根据试题所提供的信息撰写一篇约 80 词的短文。这部分考试时间为 30 分钟，分数权重为 15%。

近几年来的写作真题分为两类。一类是表格题，如 observation chart, patient record, tips to prevent deep vein thrombosis, tips to improve sleep quality, tips to prevent high blood pressure。这类表格题通常提供较为详细的患者信息，包括患者姓名、性别、年龄、住院号、出生日期、入（出）院日期、症状、体温（T）、脉搏（P）、呼吸速率（R）、血压（BP）、血氧饱和度（O_2 SATS）、医嘱、吸烟喝酒史、入院原因、家族史、过敏史等。因此，按照这类表格题写作，表格中的信息必须全部表达出来，考生将主要信息扩词成句，最后成文。一级的表格题写作比较局限，主要表达上述信息，所以考生可以多模仿范文，学会这些信息的表达。另一类是将 tips 扩充成文，考生要将这些关于疾病或保健知识的小诀窍写成一篇保健、健康宣教的文章。考生要明确写作主题，理解提供的 tips 的含义，然后按照字数要求，将 tips 表达清楚，不能有所遗漏，最好要有个总结。

学习建议：

1. 阅读

METS 一级的阅读理解在所有题型中占 55%，比例最大。以一级为例，其阅读部分共 5 项任务：信息匹配（单词等）、信息匹配（单句或告示）、补全对话、信息判断和填词补文；35

题的题量较多，分值高，权重大，所以是整个考试的重中之重。如何能够顺利完成一级的阅读题？首先要有一定的基础医学词汇储备，一级大纲的956个单词，考生在短时间内掌握所有单词需要一定的方法，可以将单词分类整理，如身体部位器官类、疾病类、症状类、医院科室类、医疗操作类等。其次考生要具备一定的阅读策略。一级考试考查了考生对医疗设备描述和医疗环境下对话的理解能力，考生必须理解关键词汇，匹配选项中的含义，这类题型难度较低，通常能理解大意就能匹配正确。一级考试阅读部分还有信息判断和填词补文题。信息判断题要求考生通读全文、明确结构、把握主题、了解细节，建议考生可以带着题干到文中寻找信息，这样比较快捷。填词补文题是全卷难度最大的，考生要理解主题、读懂词义、根据上下文、词性等确定所填之词。

2. 写作

METS一级写作题考查考生词汇、语法、逻辑思维等综合能力，是考查考生运用医学英语能力的一个重要方面。关于写作技巧和写作中应注意的问题，前面已有评述，下面再补充几点，供考生参考。

（1）关于语篇架构

一级写作要求考生写80词。有时考生容易直接书写给出的要点，不顾及文章的布局。英语中有两种规范的分段法：一种是空格不空行，即每段开头空5个字母，而每段之间不空行。第二种方法是空行不空格，即每段段首不空格，但段与段之间空一行。应该注意的是，这两种格式不能混用，即在同一篇文章中不可既有开头空格，又有段间空行。一级写作如果是tips类，那要考生自己书写开头和结尾，开头交代主题，结尾对全文做出总结，然后用first, second, third等词连接各建议。

（2）关于句子表达

一级写作要求考生准确使用医学词汇和句子表达。考生时常不注意书写完整的句子，容易直接照抄给出的信息，这样导致只有零散的词组或名词，不能形成完整的书面表达。可见，考生要练习正确句式的书写，通过理解所给的信息要点，将各信息连成具有逻辑结构的语篇文章。希望考生能阅读范文，练习书写，提高写作能力。

医护英语水平考试（一级）
模拟训练（一）

Medical English Test System（METS）Level 1
Module 1

I   Listening

Part One >>>>>>

 Questions 1—5

- You will hear five patients describing their pain. Decide where each patient has the pain.
- Write the appropriate letter **A—H** in each box.
- Mark the corresponding letter on your **answer sheet**.
- You will hear each conversation twice.

🔊 **Example:**

0.   Tim   F

---

1. Rachel   ☐   **A.** In the ankle.

2. Brian   ☐   **B.** In the back.

3. Karen   ☐   **C.** In the leg.

4. Edith   ☐   **D.** In the arm.

5. Cindy   ☐   **E.** In the finger.

                                     F. In the wrist.

                                     G. In the knee.

                                     H. In the chest.

Part Two >>>>>>

 ## Questions 6—10

- You will hear a conversation of a nurse talking to a patient.
- For each of the following sentences，decide whether it is **True**（**A**）or **False**（**B**）. Put a tick（✓）in the relevant box.
- Mark the corresponding letter on your **answer sheet**.
- You will hear the conversation twice.

Example：

0. The nurse is talking with Mr. Benson.   **A.** True   ✓

                                             B. False

---

6. Mr. Benson fell down when he was walking.   **A.** True

                                                  B. False

7. Mr. Benson hit his head.   **A.** True

                                  B. False

8. Mr. Benson has a headache now.   **A.** True

                                        B. False

9. Mr. Benson's pain is in the centre of the head.   **A.** True

                                                         B. False

10. Mr. Benson doesn't need any pain relief drug.   **A.** True

                                                        B. False

Part Three >>>>>

 Questions 11—15

- You will hear a nurse explaining an examination of the gall bladder to a patient.
- For each of the following questions (or unfinished sentences), choose the correct answer **A**, **B** or **C**. Put a tick (✓) in the relevant box.
- Mark the corresponding letter on your **answer sheet**.
- You will hear the explanation twice.

🔊 Example:

0. The patient has a/an _____.

A. abdominal pain	✓
B. chest pain	
C. stomachache	

---

11. The patient needs to have a special _____.

A. CT	
B. X-ray	
C. blood test	

12. Before examination, the patient will _____.

A. take some tablets	
B. have enough water	
C. have nothing to eat	

13. The patient will be taken pictures to see _____.

A. if the pancreas is OK	
B. if there are any stones	
C. if there is a chest pain	

14. Is it painful to have the examination?

A. Yes.	
B. No.	
C. That depends.	

15. How long does the examination take?

A. Half an hour.	
B. Twenty minutes.	
C. Five to ten minutes.	

Part Four >>>>>>

 Questions 16—20

- You will hear a nurse making a patient referral over the phone.
- Fill in the blanks.
- Write the answers on your **answer sheet**.
- You will hear the conversation twice.

	Referral
Patient Name	John (**16**)_____
Ward	6
Bed	(**17**)_____
Referral to	A Speech and Language (**18**)_____
Problems	Has difficulty (**19**)_____ after stroke and needs help with feeding
Diet	Thickened fluids
Tests	(**20**) A _____ scan at 2:00 p. m.
Appointment	At 4:00 p. m.

II   Reading and Writing

Part One >>>>>>>

 Questions 21—25

- Read the following descriptions of some medical terms.
- Match each of the following descriptions with the correct term **A—H**.
- Mark the corresponding letter on your **answer sheet**.

Example:

0. It is used to measure a patient's temperature.

Answer: | 0 | A B C D E F G H

> **A.** thermometer   **E.** oxygen mask
> **B.** dressing   **F.** walking frame
> **C.** CT scan   **G.** IV drip
> **D.** forceps   **H.** stethoscope

21. It is used to give a patient fluids and medicine through the vein.

22. It is used by a doctor to pick up or hold things.

23. It is a covering placed over a wound to help healing.

24. It is used to help disabled or injured people walk.

25. It is a procedure that takes pictures of body organs.

Part Two >>>>>>

 Questions 26—30

- Read the following notices.
- Match each notice **A—G** with the appropriate description.
- Mark the corresponding letter on your **answer sheet**.

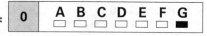 **Example：**

0. You help a patient sit up in bed with this.

Answer：

0	A	B	C	D	E	F	G
	☐	☐	☐	☐	☐	☐	■

---

26. I want to read about nursing knowledge.

27. Please don't come in the morning.

28. I can take it when I catch a cold.

29. Click here to find some job information.

30. Use it when you want to control your weight.

A. Nursingtimesjobs. com
Jobs in Nursing and Healthcare

B. Thickened Fluids Only!

C. Clinical Procedure Manual
300＋ Nursing Procedures

D. Aspirin/Pain Reliever/Fever Reducer
Runny Nose
Sore Throat
Headache＋Body Ache

E. Visiting Hours
2：00 p. m. —5：00 p. m.

F. Weight Tracker
Set your goal weight and track your progress

G. Bed Ladder Lifting Pole

Part Three　>>>>>>

 Questions 31—35

- Complete the following conversation between a nurse and a patient by filling in each blank with the appropriate sentence **A—H**.
- Mark the corresponding letter on your **answer sheet**.

Example：

Nurse：Good morning, Jane.
Patient：(**0**)＿＿＿＿＿

Answer：| 0	A B C D E F G H
	□ □ □ □ □ □ □ ■

Nurse：　How are you feeling?

Patient：(**31**)＿＿＿＿

Nurse：　What happened to you?

Patient：(**32**)＿＿＿＿

Nurse：　Where does it hurt?

Patient：(**33**)＿＿＿＿

Nurse：　Can you move your fingers?

Patient：(**34**)＿＿＿＿

Nurse：　There is a cut on your leg.　It's deep.　Is it painful?

Patient：(**35**)＿＿＿＿

Nurse：　Maybe.　I will ask the doctor to come.

Patient：Thank you.

A. Here, around my wrist.

B. Oh, I am feeling terrible.

C. Since yesterday.

D. Yes, very painful.　Will I need stitches?

E. It comes and goes.

F. I fell off my bike.

G. Yes, I can move them slowly.

H. Good morning.

Part Four >>>>>>

 Questions 36—45

- Read the following passage.
- For each of the following sentences, decide whether it is **True**（**A**）or **False**（**B**）. If there is not enough information to answer **True**（**A**）or **False**（**B**），choose **Not Given**（**C**）.
- Mark the corresponding letter on your **answer sheet**.

Save a Life! Act Now!

Studies show that fifty percent of all deaths are due to cardiovascular diseases. Sixty percent to seventy percent of these deaths occur before the victims being sent to a hospital. This means cardiovascular diseases are the first killer on the planet!

Learning CPR（Cardiopulmonary Resuscitation）allows you to save the life of a friend, a family member, or a co-worker. You can stop a sudden death caused by heart attack, stroke, or choking.

Learn CPR now! You should make sure if the surrounding scene is safe. Tell someone nearby to call 911. Check the person's breath and pulse. If the person has no breathing or pulse, begin CPR.

First, give the person mouth-to-mouth resuscitation. Support his head, lift it on back, hold his nose closed, and then open his mouth and breathe strongly into it. Give two full breaths into his mouth.

Second, turn his head. Put your hand on his chest. Put your other hand on the top of your first hand. Push downward on the chest, using the weight of your upper body for strength. Compress 15 times within 10 seconds.

Third, give two more slow breaths after the 15 compressions. Perform the 15-compression, two-breath cycle a total of four times. Re-check his pulse and breathing. Continue your performance until professional medical help arrives.

🔊 **Example:**

0. CPR means cardiopulmonary resuscitation.

A. True   **B.** False   **C.** Not Given   **Answer:** 0 | A B C |

---

36. Studies show that 60%—70% of all deaths are due to cardiovascular diseases.
A. True   **B.** False   **C.** Not Given

37. Some people had died before they were taken to hospital.
A. True   **B.** False   **C.** Not Given

38. Diabetes is the second killer in the world.
A. True   **B.** False   **C.** Not Given

39. Learning CPR helps us to save all lives.
A. True   **B.** False   **C.** Not Given

40. Heart attack, stroke and choke may cause a sudden death.
A. True   **B.** False   **C.** Not Given

41. Before performing CPR, you should check whether the surrounding area is safe.
A. True   **B.** False   **C.** Not Given

42. You need a nurse to help you when performing CPR.
A. True   **B.** False   **C.** Not Given

43. When being given mouth-to-mouth breathing, the victim opens his mouth and nose.
A. True   **B.** False   **C.** Not Given

44. You should press the chest 15 times within 10 minutes.
A. True   **B.** False   **C.** Not Given

45. CPR needs to be performed without any pause until professional medical help comes.
A. True   **B.** False   **C.** Not Given

Part Five >>>>>>

 Questions 46—55

- Read the following passage about a patient profile.
- Fill in each blank with the correct word from the list **A—L** in the box below.
- Mark the corresponding letter on your **answer sheet**.

Alan Jameson

Alan Jameson is a 53-year-old driver. He was (**46**) _____ to the hospital this morning and (**47**) _____ of the pain in his right leg and in his back. It started about eight weeks ago and it has become gradually more (**48**) _____ over the past couple of weeks. At first, he thought he'd just pulled a muscle. But it's got so bad that he hasn't been able to do his work (**49**) _____. It's also been getting to the stage when the pain is (**50**) _____ him up at night. It has been so severe, and he has noticed some tingling （麻刺感） pain (**51**) _____ his right foot. He has difficulty in carrying on with his work and loses some (**52**) _____, about three kilos. So he has become quite (**53**) _____. In the past, he suffered from intermittent pain in his back. Painkillers gave him some relief, but didn't solve the problem completely. After examination, he was (**54**) _____ numbness in his toes in the right foot. Apart from that, no other (**55**) _____ problems were reported.

A. waking	**B.** surgeon	**C.** properly
D. complained	**E.** weight	**F.** health
G. in	**H.** admitted	**I.** depressed
J. found	**K.** recover	**L.** severe

Part Six >>>>>>

 Question 56

Here are some tips to avoid falling or injury after a stroke.

Tips to avoid falling or injury after a stroke
- Clear the ways to the kitchen, bedroom and bathroom.
- Wear comfortable shoes and keep the floor dry.
- Use your walking frame even if it is a short distance.
- Don't walk in the dark.
- Take your time when walking.

- Read the tips and write a poster.
- Write the poster in about **80 words** on your **answer sheet**.

医护英语水平考试(一级)
模拟训练(二)

Medical English Test System（METS）Level 1
Module 2

Ⅰ　Listening

Part One >>>>>>

 Questions 1—5

- You will hear five patients describing their pain. Decide where each patient has the pain.
- Write the appropriate letter **A—H** in each box.
- Mark the corresponding letter on your **answer sheet**.
- You will hear each conversation twice.

Example:

0. Tim　　　　　　　　　　　　F

---

1. Mr. Green　　　　☐　　　　**A.** In the back.

　　　　　　　　　　　　　　　　B. In the stomach.

2. Bill　　　　　　　☐　　　　**C.** In the leg.

3. Mr. White　　　　☐　　　　**D.** In the hip.

4. Robert　　　　　☐　　　　**E.** In the head.

　　　　　　　　　　　　　　　　F. In the wrist.

5. Kathy　　　　　☐　　　　**G.** In the neck.

　　　　　　　　　　　　　　　　H. In the chest.

Part Two >>>>>>

 Questions 6—10

- You will hear a conversation of a nurse talking to a patient.
- For each of the following sentences，decide whether it is **True（A）** or **False（B）**. Put a tick（✓）in the relevant box.
- Mark the corresponding letter on your **answer sheet**.
- You will hear the conversation twice.

Example：

0. This dialogue takes place in a hospital. **A.** True ✓

 B. False ☐

---

6. The patient is called Lucy Cotton. **A.** True ☐

 B. False ☐

7. Mrs. Cotton was born in 1958. **A.** True ☐

 B. False ☐

8. Mrs. Cotton is a married woman. **A.** True ☐

 B. False ☐

9. Mrs. Cotton is allergic to nuts. **A.** True ☐

 B. False ☐

10. Mrs. Cotton's hospital number is 681459. **A.** True ☐

 B. False ☐

Part Three >>>>>>

 Questions 11—15

- You will hear a monologue of a nurse.
- For each of the following questions (or unfinished sentences), choose the correct answer **A**, **B** or **C**. Put a tick (✓) in the relevant box.
- Mark the corresponding letter on your **answer sheet**.
- You will hear the monologue twice.

Example:

0. The nurse specializes in _____.　**A.** renal care ✓

　　B. emergency care ☐

　　C. pediatrics ☐

---

11. Now, he's working in _____.　**A.** a transplant unit ☐

　　B. an intensive care unit ☐

　　C. a pain management unit ☐

12. He is looking after _____.　**A.** an old lady ☐

　　B. a young girl ☐

　　C. a little boy ☐

13. In his job, he doesn't like _____.　**A.** carrying out tests ☐

　　B. giving medication ☐

　　C. dealing with paper work ☐

14. In the future, he hopes to be _____　**A.** an advanced practice nurse ☐

　　B. a consultant ☐

　　C. a surgeon ☐

15. In his free time, he likes _____.　**A.** playing games ☐

　　B. climbing mountains ☐

　　C. going to the cinema ☐

Part Four >>>>>>

Questions 16—20

- You will hear a conversation of a nurse getting personal details from a patient.
- Fill in the blanks.
- Write the answers on your **answer sheet.**
- You will hear the conversation twice.

Birmingham Hospital **PATIENT RECORD**	Date & Time 9:00 21/05/12
Surname Bennett	First Name（**16**）_____
DOB 5/5/1980	Gender M
Weight	（**17**）_____kg
Temperature	（**18**）_____℃
BP	120/78
（**19**）_____	68
（**20**）_____	98％

Ⅱ　**Reading and Writing**

Part One　>>>>>>

 Questions 21—25

- Read the following descriptions of some medical terms.
- Match each of the following descriptions with the correct term **A—H**.
- Mark the corresponding letter on your **answer sheet**.

Example:

0. You use it to listen to the sounds generated inside the body.

Answer:　0　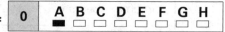

A. stethoscope	E. contrast
B. bandage	F. thermometer
C. X-ray test	G. syringe
D. heat pack	H. hand block

21. It is a medical instrument used to inject or withdraw fluids.

22. It is a test that takes a picture of the bones.

23. It is a special dye which is used to show blood vessels clearly.

24. It is used to help patients move themselves in bed.

25. It is a heated pad which soothes sore muscles.

Part Two >>>>>>

 ## Questions 26—30

- Read the following notices.
- Match each notice **A—G** with the appropriate description.
- Mark the corresponding letter on your **answer sheet**.

Example：

0. You help a patient sit up in bed with this.

Answer： | 0 | A B C D E F G |

---

26. You have to get the medicine with a doctor's prescription.

27. Click here to get a job.

28. The patients are waiting for reception here.

29. If the patient takes this medicine，he can't eat hot food or seafood.

30. This food is suitable for those with diabetes.

A. HOSPITAL WAITING AREA

B. Sugar-free food is recommended.

C. Healthcarejobsite. co. uk

D. Spicy food and seafood should be restrained or avoided during the medication.

E. Prescribed Drugs

F. Smoking and tobacco are forbidden in Alexandra Hospital.

G. Bed Ladder Lifting Pole

Part Three >>>>>>

 Questions 31—35

- Complete the following conversation between a nurse and a patient by filling in each blank with the appropriate sentence **A—H**.
- Mark the corresponding letter on your **answer sheet**.

🔊 **Example：**

Nurse：Good morning, Kyle. How are you feeling, today?
Patient：(**0**)_____

Answer：

0	A	B	C	D	E	F	G	H
	☐	☐	☐	☐	☐	☐	☐	■

Nurse：Kyle, you will be on a special diet from now on. It's a low-salt diet.

Kyle：(**31**)_____

Nurse：Because you have high blood pressure, too much salt can aggravate high blood pressure.

Kyle：(**32**)_____

Nurse：That's good. Here is a list of food you should not eat.

Kyle：(**33**)_____

Nurse：Yes. You need to check the label and look for low-sodium spices. You should eat fresh vegetables, not canned vegetables.

Kyle：(**34**)_____

Nurse：Frozen vegetables are OK. Fresh vegetables are the best.

Kyle：(**35**)_____

Nurse：You're welcome. I hope you will recover soon.

A. I did not know that garlic salt had salt in it.

B. I don't like a low-salt diet.

C. OK. I will add less salt to my food now.

D. I will follow your advice. Thank you.

E. Why do I need a special diet?

F. I think my illness is not serious.

G. I know. What about frozen vegetables?

H. Good morning. I feel much better now.

Part Four >>>>>>

 Questions 36—45

- Read the following passage.
- For each of the following sentences, decide whether it is **True**（**A**）or **False**（**B**）. If there is not enough information to answer **True**（**A**）or **False**（**B**）, choose **Not Given**（**C**）.
- Mark the corresponding letter on your **answer sheet**.

What Is Anxiety?

Anxiety is a natural human reaction that involves mind and body. It serves an important basic survival function: anxiety is an alarm system that is activated whenever a person perceives danger or threat.

When the body and mind react to danger or threat, a person feels physical sensations of anxiety—things like a faster heartbeat and breathing, tense muscless, sweaty palms, a queasy stomach, and trembling hands or legs. These sensations are part of the body's fight-flight response（逃避反应）. They are caused by a rush of adrenaline（肾上腺素）and other chemicals that prepare the body to make a quick getaway from danger. They can be mild or extreme.

The fight-flight response happens instantly when a person senses a threat. It takes a few seconds longer for the thinking part of the brain to process the situation and evaluate whether the threat is real, and if so, how to handle it. If the brain sends the all-clear signal, the fight-flight response is deactivated and the nervous system can relax.

If the mind reasons that a threat might last, feelings of anxiety might linger, keeping the person alert. Physical sensations such as rapid, shallow breathing, a pounding heart, tense muscles and sweaty palms might continue, too.

◀))) Example:

0. Anxiety is a natural human reaction that involves mind and body.

A. True   **B.** False   **C.** Not Given   **Answer:**

0	A	B	C
	■	□	□

---

36. When you are in danger, anxiety is activated.
A. True   **B.** False   **C.** Not Given

37. Anxiety is an important reaction, which may save your life in an emergency.
A. True   **B.** False   **C.** Not Given

38. When you are anxious, you may have a faster heartbeat and breathing, tense muscles, sweaty palms and feel dizzy.
A. True   **B.** False   **C.** Not Given

39. All the body's fight-flight responses are a faster heartbeat and breathing, tense muscles, sweaty palms, a queasy stomach, and trembling hands or legs.
A. True   **B.** False   **C.** Not Given

40. In addition to adrenaline, hormone also causes the body's fight-flight responses.
A. True   **B.** False   **C.** Not Given

41. The body's fight-flight response only takes a few seconds to make a judgment of the situation.
A. True   **B.** False   **C.** Not Given

42. When the all-clear signal is sent by the brain, you will be relaxed.
A. True   **B.** False   **C.** Not Given

43. The physical sensations of anxiety are always strong.
A. True   **B.** False   **C.** Not Given

44. If you keep alert for a long time, you may feel tired and won't be anxious.
A. True   **B.** False   **C.** Not Given

45. As anxiety serves an important basic survival function, you need it as much as possible.
A. True   **B.** False   **C.** Not Given

Part Five >>>>>>

 Questions 46—55

- Read the following passage about body mass index.
- Fill in each blank with the correct word from the list **A—L** in the box below.
- Mark the corresponding letter on your **answer sheet**.

Body Mass Index

Health care professionals use a measurement called body mass index(BMI 身体质量指数) to figure out if a person is overweight. BMI is a calculation that uses your (**46**) _____ and weight to (**47**) _____ how much body fat you have. After calculating your BMI，a doctor or nurse will (**48**) _____ the result on a BMI chart. The growth charts have lines for "percentiles." Like (**49**) _____ , percentiles go from 0 to 100. When your BMI is on the chart，the doctor can (**50**) _____ you with the teens the same age and (**51**) _____ as you. (**52**) _____ on where your number plots on the chart，the doctor will decide if your BMI is in the (**53**) _____ , healthy weight，overweight，or (**54**) _____ range.

Anyone who falls between the 5th percentile and the 85th percentile is a healthy weight. If someone is at or (**55**) _____ the 85th percentile line(but less than the 95th percentile)，he is overweight. If someone is over the 95th percentile line on the chart，he is in the level of obesity.

A. mark	**B**. gender	**C**. Based
D. obese	**E**. height	**F**. above
G. percentages	**H**. chart	**I**. estimate
J. district	**K**. compare	**L**. underweight

Part Six >>>>>>

 Question 56

Alexandra Hospital **Patient Record**	Date and Time 10:00　26/8/14
Surname　Green	First Name　John
DOB　10/5/1995	Gender　M
Occupation	college student
Marital Status	single
Next of Kin	father, William
Contact No.	03762 – 578921
Smoking Intake	n/a
Alcohol Intake	n/a
Reason for Admission	fell down the stairs
Family History	heart disease(mother's side)
Allergies	none

• Read the patient record and write a report.

• Write the report in about **80 words** on your **answer sheet**.

医护英语水平考试(一级)

模拟训练(三)

Medical English Test System (METS) Level 1
Module 3

Ⅰ　Listening

Part One　>>>>>>

 Questions 1—5

- You will hear five patients describing their pain. Decide where each patient has the pain.
- Write the appropriate letter **A—H** in each box.
- Mark the corresponding letter on your **answer sheet**.
- You will hear each conversation twice.

Example:

0. Tim　　　　　　　　　　F

---

1. Nancy　　　　　　　　□

2. Lena　　　　　　　　　□

3. Richard　　　　　　　□

4. Daniel　　　　　　　　□

5. Eason　　　　　　　　□

A. In the head.

B. In the throat.

C. In the abdomen.

D. In the stomach.

E. In the rib.

F. In the wrist.

G. In the leg.

H. In the back.

Part Two >>>>>>

 Questions 6—10

- You will hear a conversation of a nurse talking to a patient.
- For each of the following sentences，decide whether it is **True**（**A**）or **False**（**B**）. Put a tick（√）in the relevant box.
- Mark the corresponding letter on your **answer sheet**.
- You will hear the conversation twice.

Example：

0. The patient is called Ivan.　　　　　　　　　**A.** True　[√]

　　　　　　　　　　　　　　　　　　　　　　　　B. False　[ ]

---

6. Ivan doesn't feel well today.　　　　　　　　**A.** True　[ ]

　　　　　　　　　　　　　　　　　　　　　　　　B. False　[ ]

7. Ivan has already finished his breakfast.　　　　**A.** True　[ ]

　　　　　　　　　　　　　　　　　　　　　　　　B. False　[ ]

8. The tablet which the nurse offers is for lowering　**A.** True　[ ]

　　Ivan's blood pressure.　　　　　　　　　　　　**B.** False　[ ]

9. Ivan needs to take some antibiotics today.　　　**A.** True　[ ]

　　　　　　　　　　　　　　　　　　　　　　　　B. False　[ ]

10. The antibiotics shouldn't be taken on an empty stomach.　**A.** True　[ ]

　　　　　　　　　　　　　　　　　　　　　　　　B. False　[ ]

Part Three　>>>>>>

 Questions 11—15

- You will hear a nurse explaining the admission procedure to a patient.
- For each of the following questions (or unfinished sentences), choose the correct answer **A**, **B** or **C**. Put a tick (✓) in the relevant box.
- Mark the corresponding letter on your **answer sheet**.
- You will hear the explanation twice.

🔊 **Example：**

0. The patient has some trouble with _____.
- **A.** abdomen ✓
- **B.** chest ☐
- **C.** back ☐

---

11. The patient doesn't need to bring his/her _____.
- **A.** case history ☐
- **B.** admission notice ☐
- **C.** identity card ☐

12. The patient needs to pay the advance deposit _____.
- **A.** in cash ☐
- **B.** by card ☐
- **C.** either in cash or by card ☐

13. What examination will the patient have?
- **A.** X-ray test. ☐
- **B.** CT scan. ☐
- **C.** MRI. ☐

14. Does the patient have to go to the examination room by himself/herself?
- **A.** Yes. ☐
- **B.** No. ☐
- **C.** That depends. ☐

15. When can the patient get the examination result?
- **A.** Immediately. ☐
- **B.** Today. ☐
- **C.** The following day. ☐

Part Four >>>>>>

 ## Questions 16—20

- You will hear a patient calling to make an appointment.
- Fill in the blanks.
- Write the answers on your **answer sheet**.
- You will hear the conversation twice.

	Appointment Record
Patient Name	Justin Simpson
Date of Birth	16/04/1987
Gender	(**16**) _____
Insurance No.	(**17**) _____
Department	Department of (**18**) _____
Visiting Purpose	Pain in the (**19**) _____
Doctor's Name	Dr. Smith
Time	(**20**) _____ o'clock Wednesday afternoon

II　Reading and Writing

Part One >>>>>>

 Questions 21—25

- Read the following descriptions of some medical terms.
- Match each of the following descriptions with the correct term **A—H**.
- Mark the corresponding letter on your **answer sheet**.

◀))) Example:

0. This is a flat board which helps nurses transfer patients.

Answer: | 0 | A B C D E F G H |

A. patslide	E. monitor
B. ultrasound	F. ointment
C. ambulance	G. gurney
D. swab	H. capsule

21. It is a smooth thick substance that is put on sore skin or a wound to help it heal.

22. It is a machine used to check or record processes inside a person's body.

23. You use it to get pictures of the inside of human bodies.

24. It is a vehicle for taking patients to and from hospital.

25. It is a very small tube containing powdered or liquid medicine, which a patient swallows.

Part Two >>>>>>>

Questions 26—30

- Read the following notices.
- Match each notice **A—G** with the appropriate description.
- Mark the corresponding letter on your **answer sheet**.

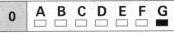 **Example：**

0. You help a patient sit up in bed with this.

Answer：

0	A	B	C	D	E	F	G
	□	□	□	□	□	□	■

---

26. You don't need to pay for them.

27. This is for any patient who has just had an abdominal surgery.

28. The patient is a two-year-old boy.

29. We offer help in emergent situations.

30. If you are interested in nursing，you can read it.

A. Help Line
84567903

B. Guidebook：
The Basic Introduction to Nursing

C. Diet after 24—72 hours of operation，waiting for intestinal function recovery.

D. For children and infants over 4 months of age，place 0.5 ml under the tongue every 20 minutes.

E. The vaccines are free of charge.

F. Registration Time
7：30—11：30
13：30—16：30

G. Bed Ladder Lifting Pole

Part Three >>>>>>

 Questions 31—35

- Complete the following conversation between a patient and a nurse with the appropriate sentence **A—H**.
- Mark the corresponding letter on your **answer sheet**.

◀)) Example:

Patient: Good morning.

Nurse: (**0**)_____

Answer: | 0 | A B C D E F G H |

Patient: I'm suffering from insomnia. It is really annoying.

Nurse: (**31**)_____

Patient: About one month.

Nurse: (**32**)_____

Patient: Yes. I tried some sleeping pills, but they didn't work.

Nurse: Do you have headaches?

Patient: (**33**)_____

Nurse: Let me take your blood pressure. You look anemic.

Patient: OK.

Nurse: Well, there is nothing to be worried about. You are just a little exhausted from overwork.

Patient: What should I do then?

Nurse: (**34**)_____

Patient: Thank you very much.

Nurse: (**35**)_____

A. Sometimes. I have a poor appetite and tend to get stressed.

B. It is hard to say.

C. Have you taken any medicine?

D. How long have you had this problem?

E. Just a moment, please.

F. You're welcome. I hope you will recover in no time.

G. I think you need more rest. Don't strain yourself too much.

H. Good morning, madam. What can I do for you?

Part Four >>>>>>

Questions 36—45

- Read the following passage.
- For each of the following sentences，decide whether it is **True（A）** or **False（B）**. If there is not enough information to answer **True（A）** or **False（B）**，choose **Not Given（C）**.
- Mark the corresponding letter on your **answer sheet**.

The Symptoms of Diabetes

From adults to children，the incidence rate of diabetes has increased everywhere in the world at an alarming frequency. When one suffers diabetes，it means that his or her cells are not getting enough glucose due to lack of insulin or due to the body cells becoming resistant to insulin.

The most common symptom of diabetes is frequent urination. The kidneys are overwhelmed by the presence of too much glucose and therefore they draw a lot of water from the kidneys to try diluting the glucose for easy passing out. This means that the bladder is filled fast and therefore you are always rushing to the toilet.

Fast weight loss is also one of the symptoms. When glucose is not taken into the cells for energy provision，the cells look for alternative ways of functioning and this leads to the breakdown of muscle in the body. It starts with the fat and after the fat is gone，the body starts eating itself，so to speak，for energy and soon，the sufferer looks weak.

Another sign of diabetic symptom is that you feel weak and tired for no reason. The reason is that the cells do not get the glucose that they are supposed to get so that they cannot provide the body with energy for their daily activities.

🔊 **Example：**

    0. There're many symptoms for diabetes.

      A. True   **B.** False   **C.** Not Given   **Answer：** | 0 | A ■ B □ C □ |

---

36. Diabetes only occurs to adults.
      A. True   **B.** False   **C.** Not Given

37. If a person is diabetic, his or her cells will get more glucose.
      A. True   **B.** False   **C.** Not Given

38. Diabetes can be divided into Type 1 and Type 2.
      A. True   **B.** False   **C.** Not Given

39. The substance which affects the glucose is called insulin.
      A. True   **B.** False   **C.** Not Given

40. Diabetes has ranked the most common disease in the world.
      A. True   **B.** False   **C.** Not Given

41. Diabetes sufferers tend to rush to toilets.
      A. True   **B.** False   **C.** Not Given

42. When glucose is taken into the cells for energy provision, the cells look for alternative ways of functioning and this leads to the breakdown of muscle in the body.
      A. True   **B.** False   **C.** Not Given

43. If you feel weak and tired for no reason, you may suffer from diabetes.
      A. True   **B.** False   **C.** Not Given

44. Some people are prone to look fat because of diabetes.
      A. True   **B.** False   **C.** Not Given

45. People have invented many new medicines to deal with diabetes.
      A. True   **B.** False   **C.** Not Given

Part Five >>>>>>

 Questions 46—55

- Read the following passage about diet products.
- Fill in each blank with the correct word from the list **A—L** in the box below.
- Mark the corresponding letter on your **answer sheet**.

Diet Products

We are surrounded by the word "diet" everywhere we look and listen. (**46**) _____ include diet Coke，diet Pepsi，diet pills，on-fat diet，vegetable diet. We have so easily been (**47**) _____ by the promise and potential of diet products that we have stopped (**48**) _____ about what diet products are doing to us. The (**49**) _____ of diet products lies not only in the psychological effects they have on us，but also (**50**) _____ the physical harm that they cause. Diet products may not be nutritional，and the chemicals that go into diet products are (**51**) _____ dangerous. Now that we are (**52**) _____ of the effects that diet products have on us，it is time to seriously think about them before we buy them. Losing weight lies in the power of minds，not in the power of chemicals. (**53**) _____ we realize this，we will be much better able to (**54**) _____ diet products，and therefore prevent the psychological and (**55**) _____ harm that comes from using them.

A. danger	**B.** resist	**C.** physical
D. attracted	**E.** in	**F.** Once
G. benefit	**H.** potentially	**I.** Examples
J. thinking	**K.** aware	**L.** from

Part Six >>>>>>

 Question 56

This is an admission form of a patient.

Admission Form		
Patient Name　Nora Hanks	Age　42	Gender　Female
Admission Time　18/07/2014	Reason for Admission　Hypertension	
Self-complaints	Headache/Vomiting in the morning	
Observations	BP	180/140 mmHg
	HR	130/min
	Res. Rate	38/min
	Temp	37.5 ℃
Nursing Instructions	1. Give anti-hypertensive drugs according to the doctor's order. 2. Offer a low-salt diet.	

- Read the information in the form.
- Write a report of the form in about **80 words** on your answer sheet.

医护英语水平考试（一级）
模拟训练（四）

Medical English Test System（METS）Level 1
Module 4

I　Listening

Part One　>>>>>>

 Questions 1—5

- You will hear five patients describing their pain. Decide where each patient has the pain.
- Write the appropriate letter **A—H** in each box.
- Mark the corresponding letter on your **answer sheet**.
- You will hear each conversation twice.

Example：

0.　Tim　　　　　　　　　　F

---

1. Sam　　　　　　　　　□　　　│　　**A.** In the arm.

　　　　　　　　　　　　　　　　　│　　**B.** In the back.

2. Judy　　　　　　　　□　　　│　　**C.** In the chest.

3. Bill　　　　　　　　□　　　│　　**D.** In the knee.

　　　　　　　　　　　　　　　　　│　　**E.** In the stomach.

4. Martin　　　　　　　□　　　│　　**F.** In the wrist.

5. Linda　　　　　　　□　　　│　　**G.** In the ankle.

　　　　　　　　　　　　　　　　　│　　**H.** In the tooth.

Part Two >>>>>>

 Questions 6—10

- You will hear a conversation between a nurse and a patient.
- For each of the following sentences，decide whether it is **True(A)** or **False(B)**. Put a tick（✓）in the relevant box.
- Mark the corresponding letter on your **answer sheet**.
- You will hear the conversation twice.

Example：

0. The patient is called Mr. Parsons.　　**A.** True　☑

　　　　　　　　　　　　　　　　　　B. False　☐

---

6. Mr. Parsons is ready to go home.　　**A.** True　☐

　　　　　　　　　　　　　　　　　　B. False　☐

7. A salt-free diet leads to Mr. Parsons' poor appetite.　**A.** True　☐

　　　　　　　　　　　　　　　　　　B. False　☐

8. Mr. Parsons shouldn't drink beer because he is too fat.　**A.** True　☐

　　　　　　　　　　　　　　　　　　B. False　☐

9. Mr. Parsons' blood pressure is not high now.　**A.** True　☐

　　　　　　　　　　　　　　　　　　B. False　☐

10. The nurse is very patient to Mr. Parsons.　**A.** True　☐

　　　　　　　　　　　　　　　　　　B. False　☐

Part Three >>>>>>

 Questions 11—15

- You will hear a monologue of a doctor talking about adult acne.
- For each of the following questions (or unfinished sentences), choose the correct answer **A, B** or **C.** Put a tick (√) in the relevant box.
- Mark the corresponding letter on your **answer sheet**.
- You will hear the monologue twice.

Example：

0. What is the patient's problem?

    A. Adult acne. ☑

    B. Cold. ☐

    C. Bad mood. ☐

---

11. The doctor is a _____.

    A. skin doctor ☐

    B. surgeon ☐

    C. dentist ☐

12. Which of the following is not the reason for acnes?

    A. Pressure. ☐

    B. Endocrine disorder. ☐

    C. Depression. ☐

13. The patient should wash face with _____.

    A. cold water ☐

    B. warm water ☐

    C. clean water ☐

14. What kind of food may cause acne?

    A. Spicy food. ☐

    B. Salty food. ☐

    C. Sour food. ☐

15. How many times should the patient use the cream?

    A. Once a day. ☐

    B. Twice a day. ☐

    C. Three times a day. ☐

Part Four >>>>>>

Questions 16—20

- You will hear a conversation between a doctor and a patient.
- Fill in the blanks.
- Write the answers on your **answer sheet**.
- You will hear the conversation twice.

Medical Record	
Surname (**16**) _____	First Name Tim
Gender	Male
Phone Number	4225329682
Symptoms	(**17**) _____, chest pain and a high fever
Temperature	(**18**) _____ ℃
Examinations	ECG and an (**19**) _____ examination
Allergies	(**20**) _____

Ⅱ　Reading and Writing

Part One >>>>>>

 Questions 21—25

- Read the following descriptions of some medical terms.
- Match each of the following descriptions with the correct term **A—H**.
- Mark the corresponding letter on your **answer sheet**.

🔊 **Example:**

0. It is a tool to help any weak or disabled person sit or move around.

Answer: | **0** | **A B C D E F G H**

A. wheelchair	**E.** retractor
B. stethoscope	**F.** scalpel
C. syringe	**G.** thermometer
D. MRI	**H.** swab

21. It is an instrument for measuring temperature.

22. It is a knife with a sharp blade used by surgeons during operations.

23. It is an instrument that a doctor uses to listen to your heart and breathing.

24. It can be used to get a picture of the soft parts inside a patient's body.

25. It is a small piece of cotton wool used by a doctor or nurse for cleaning a wound.

Part Two >>>>>>

 Questions 26—30

- Read the following notices.
- Match each notice **A—G** with the appropriate description.
- Mark the corresponding letter on your **answer sheet**.

Example：

0. You help a patient sit up in bed with this.

Answer： | 0 | A B C D E F G ▢▢▢▢▢▢■ |

---

26. You can use it only if your doctor asks you to.

27. You should not smoke in this area.

28. The patient's blood sugar is high.

29. You will be taken into this place if you have a sudden illness.

30. You should not get close to this area if not necessary.

A. Sugar-Free Diet

B. Radiation Risk

C. To Be Used under the Doctor's Supervision

D. Non-Smoking Ward

E. Emergency Room

F. Out-Patient Department

G. Bed Ladder Lifting Pole

Part Three >>>>>>

 Questions 31—35

- Complete the following conversation between a nurse and a patient by filling in each blank with the appropriate sentence **A—H**.
- Mark the corresponding letter on your **answer sheet**.

Example:

Nurse: Good morning.
Patient: (**0**)_____

Answer: | 0 | A B C D E F G H
☐ ☐ ☐ ☐ ☐ ☐ ☐ ■

Nurse: Are you here to see a doctor?

Patient: Yes. I'm not feeling well.

Nurse: (**31**)_____

Patient: No, this is the first time.

Nurse: (**32**)_____

Patient: Yes, I do. Here it is.

Nurse: Which department do you want to register with?

Patient: (**33**)_____ My tooth aches badly.

Nurse: (**34**)_____Please don't lose it and bring it whenever you come.

Patient: Yes, I will. (**35**)_____

Nurse: Go downstairs in this hall. Make a left turn at the pharmacy and you are there.

Patient: Thank you very much.

A. Can you tell me how to get to the dentist's office?

B. Do you have a registration card?

C. This is your registration card.

D. What's the matter?

E. Have you ever been here before?

F. I have a very good appetite.

G. I want to see a dentist.

H. Good morning.

Part Four >>>>>>

 Questions 36—45

- Read the following passage.
- For each of the following sentences, decide whether it is **True (A)** or **False (B)**. If there is not enough information to answer **True (A)** or **False (B)**, choose **Not Given (C)**.
- Mark the corresponding letter on your **answer sheet**.

What's Your Real Age?

Lily Cook often works out at the gym. She has a slim body, smooth skin and shiny hair. Surprisingly, despite her youthful appearance, Cook is 60 years old. Why do some people look young while others seem older than their actual age?

According to the anti-aging experts at RealAge, Inc., everyone has two ages. One is chronological age determined by birthday; the other is a real age determined by lifestyle. RealAge, Inc., a health company, uses Internet tools and other media to encourage people to look and feel years younger.

After discovering 125 factors that influence aging, such as smoking, exercise and an amount of sleep, the company created a comprehensive test to determine one's real age and help them feel younger. The online test set by the company is free. To offer you healthcare suggestions, RealAge may request detailed personal health information from you. According to your information, they will give you a personalized plan to help you feel younger and a list of what's making you younger and older. So, what is your real age? You will know the answer when you click into the company's website.

◀))) **Example：**

   0. Lily Cook often works out at the gym.

     A. True   **B.** False   **C.** Not Given   **Answer：** | 0 | A B C |

---

36. Lily Cook looks younger than her actual age.
     A. True   **B.** False   **C.** Not Given

37. Everyone has two ages according to the experts at RealAge.
     A. True   **B.** False   **C.** Not Given

38. The chronological age is determined by lifestyle.
     A. True   **B.** False   **C.** Not Given

39. RealAge, Inc. is an Internet company.
     A. True   **B.** False   **C.** Not Given

40. Smoking is a factor that may influence aging.
     A. True   **B.** False   **C.** Not Given

41. The amount of sleep has nothing to do with aging.
     A. True   **B.** False   **C.** Not Given

42. Lack of sleep will lead to aging.
     A. True   **B.** False   **C.** Not Given

43. You have to pay for the test set by RealAge, Inc.
     A. True   **B.** False   **C.** Not Given

44. In the test, you need to give your detailed personal information.
     A. True   **B.** False   **C.** Not Given

45. After finishing the test, you will be given a plan to help you feel younger.
     A. True   **B.** False   **C.** Not Given

Part Five >>>>>>

 Questions 46—55

- Read the following passage about a patient profile.
- Fill in each blank with the correct word from the list **A—L** in the box below.
- Mark the corresponding letter on your **answer sheet**.

Mr. Smith

Mr. Smith was 79 years old. He was (**46**) _____ to hospital on June 9, because of cough and chest pain for nearly 1 month, together with weakness. His (**47**) _____ got worse within 5 days. The cough got serious at night, and the patient sometimes (**48**) _____ up with it. The chest pain worsened (**49**) _____. At first, it was a needle-like pain on the right chest but it then (**50**) _____ to both sides near the lung. The pain was associated with the patient's position and (**51**) _____. The X-ray (**52**) _____ indicated a moderate amount of pleural effusion(胸腔积液). The patient came to hospital in the afternoon and was (**53**) _____ with chest drainage(胸腔引流). Since the disease came on, the patient hadn't had obvious (**54**) _____ loss. He was in normal nutritional and conscious condition. (**55**) _____ examinations were needed.

A. overweight	**B.** weight	**C.** admitted
D. spread	**E.** symptoms	**F.** movement
G. treated	**H.** woke	**I.** lifestyles
J. Further	**K.** examination	**L.** gradually

Part Six >>>>>>

 Question 56

Here is the admission record of a patient.

Admission Record	
Patient Name	Emma Roberts
DOB	Feb. 14, 1984
Gender	Female
Marital Status	Married
Contact Number	37784005279
Date of Admission	June 26, 2017
Symptoms	Headache and vomiting
Physical Examination	T: 38℃ P: 108/min R: 24/min BP: 120/80 mmHg
Further Examinations	X-ray Blood test

- Write a summary of the patient in no less than 80 words according to the record.
- Write the summary on your answer sheet.

医护英语水平考试(一级)

模拟训练(五)

Medical English Test System（METS）Level 1
Module 5

I　Listening

Part 1　>>>>>

Questions 1—5

- You will hear five patients describing their pain. Decide where each patient has the pain.
- Write the appropriate letter **A—H** in each box.
- Mark the corresponding letter on your **answer sheet**.
- You will hear each conversation twice.

Example:

0.　Tim　　　　　　　　F

---

1. Blake　　　　　□

2. Paul　　　　　□

3. Jack　　　　　□

4. Susan　　　　　□

5. Mike　　　　　□

A. In the knee.

B. In the chest.

C. In the ear.

D. In the head.

E. In the leg.

F. In the wrist.

G. In the throat.

H. In the back.

Part Two >>>>>>

 Questions 6—10

- You will hear a conversation of a nurse talking to a patient.
- For each of the following sentences，decide whether it is **True(A)** or **False（B）**. Put a tick (✓) in the relevant box.
- Mark the corresponding letter on your **answer sheet**.
- You will hear the conversation twice.

Example：

0. Paul cut his hand.   **A.** True   ✓

                                       B. False   ☐

---

6. Paul works as a builder with a knife.   **A.** True   ☐

                                       B. False   ☐

7. Paul does not have a deep cut in his hand.   **A.** True   ☐

                                       B. False   ☐

8. It is hard to heal from a knife cut.   **A.** True   ☐

                                       B. False   ☐

9. Paul needs a tetanus injection.   **A.** True   ☐

                                       B. False   ☐

10. Paul came to see the doctor because he thought   **A.** True   ☐

      his hand cut needed stitches.   **B.** False   ☐

Part Three >>>>>>

 ## Questions 11—15

- You will hear a conversation between a nurse and a patient.
- For each of the following questions (or unfinished sentences), choose the correct answer **A**, **B** or **C**. Put a tick (✓) in the relevant box.
- Mark the corresponding letter on your **answer sheet**.
- You will hear the conversation twice.

🔊 **Example：**

0. How is Gary feeling?	**A.** Much better. ✓
	B. Very bad. ☐
	C. Bitterly painful. ☐

---

11. Fever helps the body to _____.	**A.** keep warm ☐
	B. reduce the pain ☐
	C. fight against diseases ☐
12. What temperature would be fatal to human beings?	**A.** 36.5 ℃. ☐
	B. 39 ℃. ☐
	C. Above 44.5 ℃. ☐
13. Fever can be reduced by _____.	**A.** aspirin ☐
	B. a dry towel on the forehead ☐
	C. a bath ☐
14. You should go to see a doctor if a fever persists for _____.	**A.** more than five hours ☐
	B. more than five days ☐
	C. more than half a month ☐
15. A high body temperature can be brought down by drinking _____.	**A.** hot water ☐
	B. cold drinks ☐
	C. warm soup ☐

Part Four >>>>>

 Questions 16—20

- You will hear a conversation in the Outpatient Department between a nurse and a patient.
- Fill in the blanks.
- Write the answers on your **answer sheet.**
- You will hear the conversation twice.

Surname Connolly	**First Name** Wentworth
Age 30	**Gender** M
Date of Admission	(**16**) _____
Marital Status	(**17**) _____
Occupation	(**18**) _____
Hospital No.	654321
Present Complaints	(**19**) _____ in the urine High blood pressure
General Conditions	Good BP (**20**) _____ CVS HR 75/min HS normal

II Reading and Writing

Part One >>>>>>

 ## Questions 21—25

- Read the following descriptions of some medical terms.
- Match each of the following descriptions with the correct term **A—H**.
- Mark the corresponding letter on your **answer sheet**.

Example:

0. This is a chair with wheels in which someone can sit and be moved around.

Answer: | 0 | A B C D E F G H |

A. wheelchair	E. mask
B. ultrasound	F. scale
C. pipette	G. ICU
D. syringe	H. elbow

21. Very ill patients are taken into this place.

22. It is used to weigh a patient.

23. It is used to get pictures of the inside of human bodies.

24. It is a medical instrument used to inject or withdraw fluids.

25. It is the outer part of the joint where the arm bends.

Part Two ⟩⟩⟩⟩⟩⟩

 ## Questions 26—30

- Read the following notices.
- Match each notice **A**—**G** with the appropriate description.
- Mark the corresponding letter on your **answer sheet**.

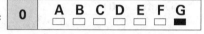 **Example：**

0. We want expert nurses.

Answer：
0	A	B	C	D	E	F	G
	□	□	□	□	□	□	■

---

26. Do not stay in the sun.

27. You can go in with a wheelchair from here.

28. You cannot smoke here.

29. You must stay away from it.

30. The patients are waiting for reception here.

A.
> WARNING
> Medical Waste

B. Avoid Sun Exposure

C. Patient Registration

D. HOSPITAL WAITING AREA

E.
> OXYGEN IN USE
> NO SMOKING

F. Disabled Ramp

G.
> Nurse Consultants
> for Elderly People
> £59,366—£71,737 p. a. inc | London

Part Three >>>>>>

 Questions 31—35

- Complete the conversation between a doctor and a patient by filling in each blank with the appropriate sentence **A—H**.
- Mark the correct letter on your **answer sheet**.

Example:

Patient: Good morning.
Doctor: (**0**)_____

Answer: | 0 | A B C D E F G H |

Patient: (**31**)_____
Doctor: How long have you had this problem?
Patient: (**32**)_____
Doctor: Have you taken any medicine?
Patient: (**33**)_____, but they have done nothing for me.
Doctor: Do you have headaches?
Patient: Sometimes. I have no appetite and am always on the edge.
Doctor: Let me take your blood pressure. (Taking the patient's blood pressure.) (**34**)_____
Patient: What should I do then?
Doctor: (**35**)_____
Patient: Thank you. I'll do as I am told.
Doctor: Here is the prescription for you. I'm sure the medicine will cure your insomnia.
Patient: Thanks a lot. Byebye!
Doctor: Bye!

A. I have tried some sleeping pills

B. I think you need more rest. Don't strain yourself too much.

C. I'm suffering from insomnia.

D. You are just a little exhausted from overwork.

E. That's good news.

F. Three months.

G. Ouch, it really hurts.

H. Good morning.

Part Four >>>>>>>

Questions 46—45

- Read the following passage.
- For each of the following sentences, decide whether it is **True (A)** or **False (B)**. If there is not enough information to answer **True (A)** or **False (B)**, choose **Not Given (C)**.
- Mark the corresponding letter on your **answer sheet**.

AIDS

The World Health Organization says as many as 10 million people worldwide may have the virus that causes AIDS. Experts believe about 350 thousand people have the disease.

There is no cure for AIDS or no vaccine to prevent it. However, researchers know much more about AIDS than they did just a few years ago. We now know that AIDS is caused by a virus. The virus invades healthy cells including white blood cells that are part of our defense system against disease. It takes control of the healthy cell's genetic(遗传的) material and forces the cell to make a copy of the virus. The cell then dies. And the viral particles move on to invade and kill more healthy cells.

The AIDS virus is carried in a person's body fluids. The virus can be passed sexually or by sharing instruments used to take intravenous drugs. It also can be passed in blood products or from a pregnant woman with AIDS to her developing baby.

Many stories about the spread of AIDS are false. You cannot get AIDS by working or attending school with someone who has the disease. You cannot get it by touching drinking glasses or other objects used by AIDS patients. Experts say no one has gotten AIDS by living with, caring for or touching an AIDS patient.

There are several warning signs of an AIDS infection. They include always feeling tired, unexplained weight loss and uncontrolled expulsion of body wastes(大小便失禁). Other warnings are the appearance of white areas in the mouth, dark red areas of skin that do not disappear and a higher than normal body temperature.

🔊 **Example：**

0. As many as 10 million people have AIDS.

A. True   **B.** False   **C.** Not Given   **Answer：** 0   A B C ■ ☐ ☐

---

36. AIDS can be prevented by some vaccine.
  A. True   **B.** False   **C.** Not Given

37. When the AIDS virus attacks our defense system, it starts to destroy our white blood cells.
  A. True   **B.** False   **C.** Not Given

38. The viral particles cannot kill healthy cells.
  A. True   **B.** False   **C.** Not Given

39. The AIDS virus does not spread through flies.
  A. True   **B.** False   **C.** Not Given

40. A person's body fluids carry the AIDS virus.
  A. True   **B.** False   **C.** Not Given

41. The AIDS virus cannot be passed from a pregnant woman to her developing baby.
  A. True   **B.** False   **C.** Not Given

42. You may get AIDS by shaking hands with a patient with the disease.
  A. True   **B.** False   **C.** Not Given

43. A nurse may get AIDS while looking after AIDS patients who are pregnant.
  A. True   **B.** False   **C.** Not Given

44. Bad headache is one of the warning signs of an AIDS infection.
  A. True   **B.** False   **C.** Not Given

45. The last paragraph is mainly talking about the possible symptoms of an AIDS infection.
  A. True   **B.** False   **C.** Not Given

Part Five >>>>>>

Questions 46—55

- Read the following passage about lung cancer.
- Fill in each blank with correct word from the list **A**—**L** in the box below.
- Mark the corresponding letter on your **answer sheet**.

Lung Cancer

It seems more people suffer from lung cancer than they did in the past. Cough is one of the (**46**)_____ for lung cancer patients. About 85 percent of men and 45 percent of women (**47**)_____ have lung cancer smoke. So obviously, lung cancer can (**48**)_____ non-smokers as well—and that is more true in women than men. Statistics show that up to 20 percent of American women (**49**)_____ with lung cancer have never smoked cigarettes. Clearly, women (**50**)_____ have a high risk of getting (**51**)_____ cancer. In fact, lung cancer in women kills more women than breast cancer. Doctors are not sure (**52**)_____ young, non-smoking women contract this disease. It could be (**53**)_____ environmental factors such as air pollution, second-hand smoke and even terrible smell from some (**54**)_____ oils. Women's lungs in general tend (**55**)_____ be larger and therefore may concentrate these poisons at higher levels in the delicate lungs.

A. affect	**B.** do	**C.** who
D. why	**E.** shift	**F.** due to
G. lung	**H.** symptoms	**I.** sure
J. cooking	**K.** to	**L.** diagnosed

Part Six >>>>>>>

 ## Question 56

This is a patient record of City Hospital.

CITY HOSPITAL	
PATIENT RECORD	**Date & Time** *10 : 00* *25 / 11 / 2017*

Surname Naton	**First Name** Robert
DOB 27/1/1967	**Gender** M
Occupation	bus driver
Marital Status	married
Next of Kin	daughter, Susan
Contact No.	4665 048 5726
Smoking Intake	n/a
Alcohol Intake	n/a
Reason for Admission	heart disease (7 years)
Family History	heart disease (father's side)
Allergies	seafood

- Write a summary of the patient in no less than 80 words according to the record.
- Write the summary on your **answer sheet**.

医护英语水平考试(一级)
模拟训练(六)

Medical English Test System (METS) Level 1
Module 6

Ⅰ   Listening

Part One >>>>>>

 Questions 1—5

- You will hear five patients describing their pain. Decide where each patient has the pain.
- Write the appropriate letter **A—H** in each box.
- Mark the corresponding letter on your **answer sheet**.
- You will hear each conversation twice.

🔊 **Example:**

0. Tim ___A___

---

1. Mr. White ☐

2. Mr. Smith ☐

3. Mr. Blaire ☐

4. Louise ☐

5. Mr. Green ☐

A. In the hand.

B. In the chest.

C. In the back.

D. In the tooth.

E. In the stomach.

F. In the wrist.

G. In the head.

H. In the throat.

Part Two >>>>>>

 Questions 6—10

- You will hear a conversation of a nurse talking to a patient.
- For each of the following sentences，decide whether it is **True**（**A**）or **False**（**B**）. Put a tick（✓）in the relevant box.
- Mark the corresponding letter on your **answer sheet**.
- You will hear the conversation twice.

Example：

| **0.** The nurse is called Mary. | **A.** True | ✓ |
| | **B.** False | ☐ |

| **6.** Mr. Gates had a pain in the head two weeks ago. | **A.** True | ☐ |
| | **B.** False | ☐ |

| **7.** Mr. Gates can't rest well at night. | **A.** True | ☐ |
| | **B.** False | ☐ |

| **8.** Mr. Gates doesn't take any painkiller for his headache. | **A.** True | ☐ |
| | **B.** False | ☐ |

| **9.** The pain is on the left side of Mr. Gates's head. | **A.** True | ☐ |
| | **B.** False | ☐ |

| **10.** The pain usually lasts for more than half an hour each time. | **A.** True | ☐ |
| | **B.** False | ☐ |

Part Three >>>>>

 Questions 11—15

- You will hear a conversation between a patient and a chemist about taking medicine.
- For each of the following questions (or unfinished sentences), choose the correct answer **A, B** or **C.** Put a tick (✓) in the relevant box.
- Mark the corresponding letter on your **answer sheet.**
- You will hear the conversation twice.

Example:

0. The chemist is talking to a _____.

    A. patient   ✓

    B. nurse   ☐

    C. doctor   ☐

---

11. It seems Mr. Brown is getting _____.

    A. a stomachache   ☐

    B. a cough   ☐

    C. a flu   ☐

12. What other symptom does Mr. Brown have?

    A. Toothache.   ☐

    B. Dizziness.   ☐

    C. Headache.   ☐

13. What medicine does the chemist suggest Mr. Brown to take?

    A. Cough mixture.   ☐

    B. Painkillers.   ☐

    C. Both A & B.   ☐

14. Mr. Brown mustn't take _____ painkillers within one day.

    A. fewer than eight   ☐

    B. more than eight   ☐

    C. eight   ☐

15. Mr. Brown will take one or two spoonfuls of the cough mixture _____.

    A. every four hours   ☐

    B. each hour   ☐

    C. every three hours   ☐

Part Four >>>>>>

 ## Questions 16—20

- You will hear a conversation between a nurse and a patient.
- Fill in the blanks.
- Write the answers on your **answer sheet**.
- You will hear the conversation twice.

Appointment Record	
Surname　Reed	**First Name**（**16**）_____
Gender	M
Purpose of Calling	Make an appointment to see the doctor for his（**17**）_____
Telephone Number	（**18**）_____
Date of Birth	the 3rd of（**19**）_____ , 1970
Visiting Time	（**20**）_____ afternoon

Ⅱ   Reading and Writing

Part One >>>>>>

 Questions 21—25

- Read the following descriptions of some medical terms.
- Match each of the following descriptions with the correct term **A—H**.
- Mark the corresponding letter on your **answer sheet**.

Example：

0. It is a tool to help any weak or disabled person sit or move around.

Answer： | **0** | A B C D E F G H

> **A.** wheelchair   **E.** operating room
> **B.** syringe   **F.** dressing
> **C.** X-ray   **G.** ambulance
> **D.** thermometer   **H.** medical chart

21. It is a vehicle used to transport seriously ill patients or injured people to hospital.

22. It is a place where surgical operations are carried out.

23. It is a document of a patient's medical history, including test results, medical orders, etc.

24. It is used to cover the wounds for patients.

25. It is a device that measures temperature.

Part Two　≫≫≫≫≫

 ## Questions 26—30

- Read the following notices.
- Match each notice **A— G** with the appropriate description.
- Mark the corresponding letter on your **answer sheet**.

Example：

0. You can visit a patient during this period.

Answer：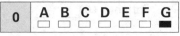

---

26. You can go there and have your teeth checked.

27. You can get different kinds of medicine there.

28. It should be put in a high place.

29. You can measure your blood pressure with it at home.

30. Take one tablet half an hour before meals.

A. Keep Out Of Reach Of Children

B. Home Testing Kit

C. Dental Centre

D. Donor Card

E. The Chemist's

F. Directions for Use：Adult Dosage

G. Visiting Hours：3:00 p. m. ～6:00 p. m.

Part Three >>>>>>

 Questions 31—35

- Complete the following conversation between a nurse and a patient by filling in each blank with the appropriate sentence **A—H**.
- Mark the corresponding letter on your **answer sheet**.

Example:

Nurse: Good morning, Mr. Hudson.
Patient: (**0**)_____

Answer: | 0 | A B C D E F G H |

Nurse: I'm Susan. What can I do for you?

Patient: Susan, I had my routine blood tests yesterday morning. When could I get the results?

Nurse: (**31**) _____

Patient: Before my operation, what should I do?

Nurse: (**32**) _____

Patient: You know, I've never had any operation before. (**33**) _____

Nurse: Just take it easy. (**34**) _____

Patient: OK. When will I have my operation?

Nurse: (**35**) _____

Patient: Oh, I know. Thank you very much.

A. You should eat properly and get enough sleep.

B. I don't know what's wrong with me.

C. Please don't hesitate to tell him.

D. Oh, you could get the results this afternoon.

E. So I'm a little bit scared.

F. The doctor and nurses will help you.

G. The day after tomorrow.

H. Good morning.

Part Four >>>>>>

Questions 36—45

- Read the following passage.
- For each of the following sentences, decide whether it is **True (A)** or **False (B)**. If there is not enough information to answer **True (A)** or **False (B)**, choose **Not Given (C)**.
- Mark the corresponding letter on your **answer sheet**.

Diabetes

Diabetes is a chronic, metabolic disease characterized by elevated levels of blood sugar, which leads over time to serious damage to the heart, blood vessels, eyes, kidneys, and nerves. Diabetes occurs when the pancreas(胰腺) does not produce enough insulin, or when the body cannot effectively use the insulin it produces. This leads to high blood sugar levels over a prolonged period. Symptoms of high blood sugar include frequent urination, increased thirst, and increased hunger.

There are three main types of diabetes. Type 1 diabetes, once known as insulin-dependent or childhood-onset diabetes, is characterized by a lack of insulin production. The cause is unknown. The most common is type 2 diabetes, usually in adults, which occurs when the body becomes resistant to insulin or doesn't produce enough insulin. It is caused by the body's ineffective use of insulin. It often results from overweight and not enough exercise. In the past three decades the prevalence of type 2 diabetes has risen dramatically in countries of all income levels. Gestational diabetes(孕期糖尿病) is the third main form and occurs when pregnant women without a previous history of diabetes develop high blood-sugar levels.

For people living with diabetes, access to affordable treatment, including insulin, is critical to their survival. There is a globally agreed target to stop the rise in diabetes and obesity by 2025.

🔊 **Example:**

0. Diabetes is a chronic disease.

A. True   **B.** False   **C.** Not Given   **Answer:** | 0 | A ■ B ☐ C ☐ |

---

36. One of the characteristics of diabetes is the elevated level of blood sugar.
A. True   **B.** False   **C.** Not Given

37. Diabetes will cause serious damage to the heart, blood vessels, eyes, kidneys, lungs and nerves.
A. True   **B.** False   **C.** Not Given

38. Symptoms of diabetes include frequent urination, increased thirst and increased hunger.
A. True   **B.** False   **C.** Not Given

39. One cause of type 1 diabetes is that the pancreas produces too much insulin.
A. True   **B.** False   **C.** Not Given

40. Overweight and not enough exercise often lead to type 2 diabetes.
A. True   **B.** False   **C.** Not Given

41. Type 2 diabetes is caused by the body's ineffective use of insulin.
A. True   **B.** False   **C.** Not Given

42. In the past three decades, type 2 diabetes has grown dramatically in the countries of all income levels.
A. True   **B.** False   **C.** Not Given

43. Gestational diabetes happens when pregnant women with a previous history of diabetes develop high blood-sugar levels.
A. True   **B.** False   **C.** Not Given

44. To keep away from diabetes, we should eat healthily, be physically active, and avoid excessive weight gain.
A. True   **B.** False   **C.** Not Given

45. A globally agreed target is to stop the rise in diabetes and obesity by 2025.
A. True   **B.** False   **C.** Not Given

Part Five >>>>>>

 Questions 46—55

- Read the following passage.
- Fill in each blank with the correct word from the list **A—L** in the box below.
- Mark the corresponding letter on your **answer sheet**.

Obesity

Obesity is a growing global health problem. Sometimes，people are so (**46**)_____ that obesity threatens their health. It typically (**47**)_____ from over-eating（especially an unhealthy diet）and lack of (**48**)_____ exercise. In our modern world with increasingly cheap，high calorie food（for example，fast food or junk food），prepared foods that are (**49**)_____ in things like salt，sugar or fat，combined with our increasingly sedentary(静态的) (**50**)_____ and changing modes of transportation，it is no wonder that obesity has (**51**)_____ increased in the last few years around the world.

Childhood obesity is also an increasing (**52**)_____ around the world. The problem of childhood obesity is (**53**)_____ many low-and middle-income countries. Globally，in 2010，the number of overweight children under the age of five was over 42 million. Nearly 35 million of them were (**54**)_____ in developing countries.

Overweight and obese children are (**55**)_____ to stay obese into adulthood and more likely to develop diseases like diabetes and cardiovascular(心血管的) diseases at a younger age.

A. overweight	**B**. likely	**C**. results
D. rapidly	**E**. enough	**F**. concern
G. living	**H**. lack	**I**. lifestyles
J. affecting	**K**. harmful	**L**. high

Part Six >>>>>>

 Question 56

Here are some tips that can help people protect their eyes.

Tips on Protecting Eyes

- Get an eye examination done at least every two years.
- Use eye drops properly.
- Watch less TV, use mobile phone less and be careful when reading.
- Get more sleep and get the right nutrition.

- Read the tips and write guidelines to help people protect their eyes.
- You are to write the guidelines in **no less than 80 words** on your **answer sheet**.

▲▲▲▲▲▲

医护英语水平考试(一级)
模拟训练(七)

Medical English Test System(METS)Level 1
Module 7

◢◢◢◢◢◢

I　Listening

Part One >>>>>>

 ### Questions 1—5

- You will hear five patients describing their pain. Decide where each patient has the pain.
- Write the appropriate letter **A—H** in each box.
- Mark the corresponding letter on your **answer sheet**.
- You will hear each conversation twice.

Example:

0. Tim　　　　　　　　　F

---

1. Terry

2. Joseph

3. Clare

4. Tina

5. Sammy

A. In the hands.

B. In the throat.

C. In the stomach.

D. In the lower back.

E. In the knee.

F. In the wrist.

G. In the ankle.

H. In the head.

Part Two >>>>>>

 Questions 6—10

- You will hear a conversation of a nurse talking to a patient.
- For each of the following sentences，decide whether it is **True**（**A**）or **False**（**B**）. Put a tick（✓）in the relevant box.
- Mark the corresponding letter on your **answer sheet**.
- You will hear the conversation twice.

Example：

0. Usha doesn't want to talk about her illness.

A. True ☐

B. False ✓

---

6. Usha enjoys her meals.

A. True ☐

B. False ☐

7. Usha's pain is getting worse.

A. True ☐

B. False ☐

8. Usha had the radiotherapy treatment.

A. True ☐

B. False ☐

9. Usha felt sick after the radiotherapy treatment.

A. True ☐

B. False ☐

10. Usha is going to have a rest.

A. True ☐

B. False ☐

Part Three >>>>>>

 ## Questions 11—15

- You will hear a conversation between a nurse and a patient.
- For each of the following questions (or unfinished sentences), choose the correct answer **A**, **B** or **C**. Put a tick (✓) in the relevant box.
- Mark the corresponding letter on your **answer sheet**.
- You will hear the conversation twice.

Example:

0. Angela is here to _____.

    A. do the dressing   ✓

    B. have a meal   ☐

    C. take a walk   ☐

---

11. First, Angela will take off the _____.

    A. clothes   ☐

    B. mask   ☐

    C. bandage   ☐

12. Mr. Briggs thinks the wound still looks _____.

    A. wonderful   ☐

    B. awful   ☐

    C. interesting   ☐

13. The skin around the wound is _____.

    A. inflamed   ☐

    B. less red   ☐

    C. perfect   ☐

14. The wound is a bit _____.

    A. larger   ☐

    B. worse   ☐

    C. smaller   ☐

15. Mr. Briggs wants to _____.

    A. watch TV   ☐

    B. have a shower   ☐

    C. have a rest   ☐

Part Four >>>>>>

 Questions 16—20

- You will hear a conversation between two nurses.
- Fill in the blanks.
- Write the answers on your **answer sheet**.
- You will hear the conversation twice.

ALEXANDRA HOSPITAL	Date & Time
INTRAVENOUS INFUSION	9 : 00 15 / 10 / 09
Before we start,	we need to wash our (**16**) _____ .
First, we will	check the IV (**17**) _____ against the IV prescription.
Next, we need to	prime the (**18**) _____ .
Then, we will	set the (**19**) _____ on the infusion pump.
The last thing is to	write up the Fluid Balance (**20**) _____ .

II   Reading and Writing

Part One   >>>>>>

 ### Questions 21—25

- Read the descriptions of pain reliefs.
- Match each of the following descriptions with the correct term **A—H**.
- Mark the corresponding letter on your **answer sheet**.

Example：

0. A heated pad soothes sore muscles.

Answer：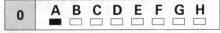

| 0 | A | B | C | D | E | F | G | H |

> **A.** heat pack   **E.** massage
>
> **B.** acupuncture   **F.** hot compress bag
>
> **C.** painkiller   **G.** syringe driver
>
> **D.** aromatherapy   **H.** ice pack

21. It is an instrument that gives a patient a continuous dose of medication.

22. Fragrant oils are used for well-being.

23. Parts of the body are rubbed or pressed to relieve pain.

24. It is a medication taken orally or by injection to stop pain.

25. Fine needles are used to relieve pain.

Part Two >>>>>>

 Questions 26—30

- Read the following notices.
- Match each notice **A—G** with the appropriate description.
- Mark the corresponding letter on your **answer sheet**.

Example:

0. Take all of the medication.

Answer: 0 A B C D E F G

---

26. Mix the contents.

27. Clean the mouth with a mouthful of water.

28. Do not stay in the sun.

29. Don't drink alcohol.

30. Throw away what is left in the container.

A. Avoid Sun Exposure

B. Avoid Alcoholic Beverages

C. Rinse Mouth with Water

D. Shake Well

E. Take on an Empty Stomach

F. Discard Contents

G. Complete the Course of Medication

Part Three >>>>>>

 Questions 31—35

- Complete the conversation between a nurse and a patient by filling in each blank with the appropriate sentence **A—H**.
- Mark the correct letter on your **answer sheet**.

Example：

Debbie：Hello, Mr. Gimlet. I have got your lunch for you.

Mr. Gimlet：(**0**)_____

Answer： 0   A B C D E F G H
                  □ □ □ □ □ □ □ ■

Debbie：	Do you have any trouble feeding yourself?	**A.** How time flies!
Mr. Gimlet：	(**31**)_____	**B.** Could you give them to me now?
Debbie：	Take your time. How could I help you?	
Mr. Gimlet：	(**32**)_____	**C.** What about the cup in your left hand?
Debbie：	Oh, I just forgot. The OT sent a few things to help you feed yourself this morning.	**D.** I need a special bowl.
		E. It looks different.
Mr. Gimlet：	(**33**)_____	**F.** Oh, that's a good idea.
Debbie：	OK. Here is a special bowl for you to try.	**G.** Yes. Sometimes I just can't hold the bowl properly.
Mr. Gimlet：	(**34**)_____	
Debbie：	It's a non-slip bowl.	
Mr. Gimlet：	(**35**)_____	**H.** Thank you, Debbie.
Debbie：	It's a non-slip cup for you.	
Mr. Gimlet：	Thank you very much.	

Part Four >>>>>>

Questions 36—45

- Read the following passage.
- For each of the following sentences，decide whether it is **True（A）** or **False（B）**. If there is not enough information to answer **True（A）** or **False（B）**，choose **Not Given（C）**.
- Mark the corresponding letter on your **answer sheet**.

A Mammogram

A mammogram(乳房 X 线检查) is an X-ray of the breast. Mammograms can be used to check for the breast cancer in women who have no signs or symptoms of the disease. This type of mammogram is called a screening mammogram(筛查性乳房 X 光检查). Screening mammograms usually involve two X-rays of each breast. They make it possible to detect tumors that cannot be felt by the patients themselves. Screening mammograms can also find micro-calcifications(微钙化) that sometimes indicate the presence of breast cancer.

Mammograms can also be used to check for breast cancer after a lump or another sign or symptom of breast cancer has been found. This type of mammogram is called a diagnostic mammogram(诊断性乳房 X 光检查). Signs of breast cancer may include pain, skin thickening, nipple discharge, or a change in breast size or shape.

Diagnostic mammograms take longer than screening mammograms because they involve more X-rays in order to obtain views of the breast from several angles. The technician may magnify(放大) an area to produce a detailed picture that can help the doctor make an accurate diagnosis.

Getting a high quality screening mammogram and having a clinical breast exam on a regular basis are the most effective ways to detect breast cancer early. As with any screening test，screening mammograms have both benefits and limitations. For example, some cancers cannot be found by a screening mammogram but may be found by a clinical breast exam.

Checking one's own breasts for lumps or other unusual changes is called a breast self-exam，or BSE. Breast self-exams cannot replace regular screening mammograms or clinical breast exams. Breast self-exams alone have not been found to help reduce the number of deaths from breast cancer.

🔊)) **Example：**

0. A mammogram is an X-ray of the breast.

   A. True   **B.** False   **C.** Not Given   **Answer：** | 0 | A B C |

---

36. Screening mammograms are used to check for breast cancer after a lump or another sign or symptom of breast cancer has been found.
   A. True   **B.** False   **C.** Not Given

37. Screening mammograms take longer than diagnostic mammograms.
   A. True   **B.** False   **C.** Not Given

38. Diagnostic mammograms usually involve more X-rays than screening mammograms.
   A. True   **B.** False   **C.** Not Given

39. Screening mammograms can find breast cancer more accurately than a clinical breast exam.
   A. True   **B.** False   **C.** Not Given

40. BSE alone can help reduce the number of deaths from breast cancer.
   A. True   **B.** False   **C.** Not Given

41. Most women choose screening mammograms for breast checking.
   A. True   **B.** False   **C.** Not Given

42. BSE can replace regular screening mammograms or clinical breast exams.
   A. True   **B.** False   **C.** Not Given

43. Diagnostic mammograms have both benefits and limitations.
   A. True   **B.** False   **C.** Not Given

44. In order to make a more accurate diagnosis, the technician may magnify an area to produce a detailed picture.
   A. True   **B.** False   **C.** Not Given

45. Signs of breast cancer may include nipple discharge or a change of breast size of shape.
   A. True   **B.** False   **C.** Not Given

Part Five >>>>>

 Questions 46—55

- Read the following passage about how to manage embarrassing moments.
- Fill in each blank with correct word from the list **A—L** in the box below.
- Mark the corresponding letter on your **answer sheet**.

How to Manage Embarrassing Moments

Some patients may always need help from doctors and nurses. They need help with daily (**46**)_____ such as having a shower or going to the toilet. Some of them can be (**47**)_____ for patients. When a patient is incontinent of (**48**)_____, he or she may feel ashamed. He or she possibly does not want to ring the (**49**)_____ for the nurse. It is always (**50**)_____ to help patients in a sensitive way so that patients do not feel embarrassed at all. Nurses should make (**51**)_____ that patients have privacy(隐私) when they are in the toilet. When nurses speak to patients，particularly elderly (**52**)_____, they should never talk down to them. It is not (**53**)_____ to look down upon patients if they have been incontinent. Above all，it's important to give patients (**54**)_____ time and not to be impatient. Nurses should know how to (**55**)_____ these moments when they work.

A. round	**B.** call bell	**C.** manage
D. patients	**E.** early	**F.** sure
G. activities	**H.** embarrassing	**I.** important
J. enough	**K.** acceptable	**L.** urine

Part Six >>>>>

 Question 56

- Read the patient record.

Alexandra Hospital **PATIENT RECORD**	**Date & Time** 15 : 00 28/12/13

Surname	Boone	**First Name**	James
DOB	3/1/82	**Gender**	M
Occupation		engineer	
Marital Status		single	
Next of Kin		Father David	
Contact No.		01863 – 652984	
Smoking Intake		n/a	
Alcohol Intake		n/a	
Reason for Admission		car accident	
Family History		heart disease (mother's side)	
Allergies		shellfish	

- Write a summary of the patient in **no less than 80 words** according to the record.
- Write the summary on your **answer sheet**.

听力文本、参考答案及解析

医护英语水平考试(一级)
模拟训练(一)

听力文本

This is METS-1 listening test. There are four parts to the test, parts One, Two, Three, and Four. You will hear each part twice. Now, look at the instructions for Part One. You will hear five patients describing their pain. Decide where each patient has the pain. Write the appropriate letter A—H in each box. Mark the corresponding letter on your answer sheet. You will hear each conversation twice.

Here is an example:

Nurse (Woman): What's brought you here, Tim?
Patient (Man): My wrist is throbbing since I fell in the street.

The answer is in the wrist, so write letter F in the box. Now we are ready to start.

Conversation 1

Nurse (Man): What happened to you, Rachel?
Patient (Woman): I fell down the stairs and broke my leg.

Conversation 2

Nurse (Woman): What's brought you here, Brian?
Patient (Man): I cut my finger when cooking. It's bleeding.

Conversation 3

Nurse (Woman): Good morning, Karen. What can I do for you?
Patient (Man): I sprained my ankle when I climbed the mountain yesterday.

Conversation 4

Nurse (Man): Are you all right, Edith?

1

Patient (Woman): No. I have some trouble with my knee. And it hurts when I'm walking.

Conversation 5

Nurse (Man): What's troubling you, Cindy?
Patient (Woman): I've got a pain in my chest.

This is the end of Part One. Now look at Part Two. You will hear a conversation of a nurse talking to a patient. For each of the following sentences, decide whether it is True (A) or False (B). Put a tick (√) in the relevant box. Mark the corresponding letter on your answer sheet. You will hear the conversation twice.

Nurse (Woman): Good morning, Mr. Benson. What's the problem?
Patient (Man): I slipped and fell down when I was having a bath.
Nurse (Woman): Then, what happened?
Patient (Man): I hit my head and saw stars at first. Now I have a headache.
Nurse (Woman): What kind of pain is it?
Patient (Man): It's a throbbing pain.
Nurse (Woman): Could you tell me where it is?
Patient (Man): In the forehead, right between my eyes.
Nurse (Woman): Is it getting a bit worse?
Patient (Man): Yes, a little bit. Could I have some pain relief drug?
Nurse (Woman): Oh, yes. I will help you have some gas and air first.
Patient (Man): Thanks.

This is the end of Part Two. Now look at Part Three. You will hear a nurse explaining an examination of the gall bladder to a patient. For each of the following questions (or unfinished sentences), choose the correct answer A, B or C. Put a tick (√) in the relevant box. Mark the corresponding letter on your answer sheet. You will hear the explanation twice.

Nurse (Woman): Good morning, sir. Since you've had an abdominal pain after fatty foods, you may have some stones in your gall bladder. You'll need to have a special X-ray done. And it will involve you taking some tablets before attending the X-ray department. They'll take an ordinary X-ray film first and then give you something fatty to eat. After that, they'll take pictures of your gall bladder area to see if it is working properly and if there are any stones. Then, they will use a special machine to examine your abdomen. The machine can show us the pictures of your

2

stomach and gall bladder. It's called ultrasonograph. It's not painful at all and it doesn't take more than five to ten minutes to perform. Do you have any questions?

This is the end of Part Three. Now look at Part Four. You will hear a nurse making a patient referral over the phone. Fill in the blanks. Write the answers on your answer sheet. You will hear the conversation twice.

Therapist（Man）：Rehab department. This is Carl speaking. Can I help you?

Nurse（Woman）：Hello. It's Lucy calling from Ward 6, Inpatient Department. I'd like to make a referral to the Speech and Language Therapist, please.

Therapist（Man）：Sure. I'm the Speech and Language therapist.

Nurse（Woman）：Right. I'm calling about patient John Hunter in bed 605.

Therapist（Man）：OK. Ward 6, bed 605. Could you spell the patient's name?

Nurse（Woman）：Of course. John, J-O-H-N, Hunter, H-U-N-T-E-R.

Therapist（Man）：Well. What's his problem?

Nurse（Woman）：He has some difficulty swallowing after stroke. And he needs help with feeding.

Therapist（Man）：I see. What type of diet is he on now?

Nurse（Woman）：He's still having thickened fluids. Could you come and see him?

Therapist（Man）：Sure. I can go and see him at 2:00 p. m. this afternoon. Is it OK?

Nurse（Woman）：Wait a minute. Let me check his notes.

Therapist（Man）：OK.

Nurse（Woman）：I'm afraid Mr. Hunter will have a CT scan at 2:00 p. m. this afternoon.

Therapist（Man）：Would 4:00 p. m. be OK?

Nurse（Woman）：Yes, that would be better.

Therapist（Man）：All right. I'll be there at 4:00 p. m.

Nurse（Woman）：See you at 4:00. Bye.

This is the end of Part Four. You now have five minutes to write your answers on the answer sheet. You have one more minute. This is the end of the listening test.

参考答案及解析

I Listening Test

Part One

听力测试第一部分是信息匹配题。此部分检测考生是否已经掌握人类身体部位的相关医学英语词汇。考生听取护士与患者之间的对话后，理解患者对受伤部位或疼痛部位的描述，并对患者姓名和他们的伤痛部位进行信息匹配。

1. C 本题中，患者 Rachel 描述自己下楼梯跌倒，并摔断了腿（leg），故选 C In the leg。

2. E 本题中，患者 Brian 告诉护士，他做菜时切伤了手指（finger），手指正在流血，故选 E In the finger。

3. A 本题中，患者 Karen 跟护士说，他昨天爬山时扭伤（sprain）了脚踝（ankle），故选 A In the ankle。

4. G 本题中，患者 Edith 提及，她走路时膝盖(knee)疼痛，故选 G In the knee。

5. H 本题中，患者 Cindy 自述胸部(chest)疼痛，故选 H In the chest。

Part Two

听力测试第二部分是信息判断题。考生听完护士对患者入院情况的询问后，根据患者所描述的病情信息，考生对所给的信息进行分析、判断。此部分的信息量较大，因此考生应按照题目顺序，完成作答。

6. B 患者描述在洗澡时摔倒，而不是在走路时摔倒，故选 B。

7. A 患者摔倒时撞到头部，起初他眼冒金星（see stars），故选 A。

8. A 患者现在的症状是头痛（headache），故选 A。

9. B 患者疼痛的部位在额头（in the forehead），而不是在头中心，故选 B。

10. B 患者要求使用缓解疼痛的药物（pain relief drug），护士同意，故选 B。

Part Three

听力测试第三部分是医护人员向患者解释将要进行的胆囊（gall bladder）影像检查。考生听完后，要根据题干给出的信息和已经听到的内容，选择正确的答案。在答题时，考生应该关注题干的重点信息。

11. B 护士提到患者腹部疼痛，需要做胆囊 X 光检查，故选 B X-ray。

12. A 护士提到患者检查前要先服用一些药片，故选 A take some tablets。

13. B 护士告知患者拍摄影像片子是为了确认胆囊是否正常工作和是否存在结石，故选 B if there are any stones。

14. B 护士提到这项检查没有疼痛，故选 B No。

15. C 护士说该项检查时间五到十分钟，故选 C Five to ten minutes。

Part Four

听力测试第四部分是护士与言语治疗师之间关于病人转诊的预约电话。考生在听的过程中，需要理解表格中的各项信息，抓住预约电话中的关键词，填写听到的有关患者的信息。

16. Hunter 听力原文中患者的姓名是 John Hunter,故填入姓 Hunter。

17. 605 听力原文中两次提到患者床号为 605,故填 605。

18. therapist 听力原文中提到患者需要言语治疗师(Speech and Language therapist)并进行转诊治疗,故填 therapist。

19. swallowing 听力原文中提到患者中风后吞咽有困难,故填 swallowing。

20. CT 听力原文中提到患者下午两点要做 CT 检查(CT scan),故填 CT。

Ⅱ Reading and Writing

Part One

阅读和写作测试的第一部分是医院中常见物品、器械和基本的诊疗技术名称与其定义的匹配。此部分主要考查考生是否掌握了常见的医疗物品或器械的英语词汇。要求考生作答时,理解每一条定义和每一个物品或器械的名称,并进行匹配。

21. G 该技术用于给患者静脉补液或给药。IV drip:静脉滴注。故选 G。

22. D 医生用该器械夹起或夹住物品。forceps:镊子。故选 D。

23. B 该物品用于覆盖伤口并帮助愈合。dressing:敷料。故选 B。

24. F 该器械用于帮助残伤人士行走。walking frame:助行架。故选 F。

25. C 该操作拍摄人体器官的照片。CT scan:电脑断层扫描。故选 C。

Part Two

阅读和写作测试的第二部分是信息匹配题,主要考查考生理解简短信息的能力。要求考生将信息告示栏与相应的简短语言描述进行匹配。答题时,考生应关注关键词,并理解信息,进行正确的匹配。

26. C 本题题干:我想阅读有关护理的知识。按照常识,能够阅读的东西有书籍、手册等。C:临床操作手册 300+护理操作程序。故选 C。

27. E 本题题干:请不要在早晨来。E:探视时间下午 2:00—5:00,符合题干要求。故选 E。

28. D 本题题干:感冒时我可以服用它。D:阿司匹林(aspirin),镇痛(pain reliever),解热(fever reducer),消除流涕(runny nose),咽喉痛(sore throat),头痛(headache),身体疼痛(body ache)。故选 D。

29. A 本题题干:点击这里,找到一些工作信息。A:医护就业的网址,符合题干要求。故选 A。

30. F 本题题干:当你想要控制体重时,使用它。F:重量跟踪器检测仪,设定目标体重,跟踪你的进展。故选 F。

Part Three

阅读和写作测试的第三部分是补全对话。主要考查考生理解护士与患者之间常见对话的能力。要求考生根据护士的问题从选项中选择正确的患者回答。注意:选项中有两项是多余信息,请仔细辨别。

31. B 对话中,护士问患者感觉如何,在选项中找出表达感觉的句子有 B 和 D,但是 D 选项提及"缝合"(stitch),与上下文不符。故选 B。

32. F 对话中,护士问患者发生了什么,只有 F 选项表达了患者"我从自行车上摔了下来"。故选 F。

33. A　对话中,护士问患者哪里受伤了,考生要从选项中找到有关身体部位的词,A 选项:手腕周围(around my wrist)。故选 A。

34. G　对话中,护士问患者手指能动吗,患者回答能慢慢动,故选 G。

35. D　对话中,护士注意到患者腿上有一处割伤,问患者疼不疼,患者回答伤口很疼,并问是否要"缝合"(stitch)。故选 D。

Part Four

阅读和写作测试的第四部分是信息判断题。考生阅读一篇关于心肺复苏操作的说明文章,要求理解何时进行 CPR(Cardiopulmonary Resuscitation),如何操作 CPR。答题时,考生需要认真阅读、判断信息,将题目与原文中信息进行比较,并做出"对""错"或"未提及"的选择。

36. B　题干:研究表明 60%—70% 的死亡是由心血管疾病造成的。文章中第一段第一句:研究表明 50% 的死亡是由心血管疾病造成的。故选 B。

37. A　题干:一些人被送到医院之前就已经死亡。文章中第一段第二句:60% 到 70% 的死亡在患者被送达医院之前发生。故选 A。

38. C　题干:糖尿病是第二杀手。文章第一段最后一句:心血管疾病是这个星球的一号杀手。其后并没有说第二位的死亡原因是什么,所以不能确定糖尿病是第二杀手。故选 C。

39. B　题干:学习心肺复苏可以拯救所有人的生命。文章第二段认为,"学习心肺复苏可以拯救我们的朋友、家人或同事"。题干中"all"覆盖的面太广,错了。故选 B。

40. A　题干:心脏病、中风和窒息会引起突发死亡。文章第二段最后一句:你可以阻止由心脏病、中风和窒息引起的突发死亡。故选 A。

41. A　题干:在进行心肺复苏(CPR)之前应该查看周围环境是否安全。文章第三段第二句表明相同的意思,故选 A。

42. C　题干:你需要一名护士协助你完成 CPR。文章没有表达这个意思,故选 C。

43. B　题干:口对口人工呼吸时,患者的口鼻要张开。文章第四段表明,口对口人工呼吸需要捏住鼻子。故选 B。

44. B　题干:在 10 分钟内按压胸部 15 次。文章第五段最后一句表明,在 10 秒内按压胸部 15 次。题干的"minutes"与文章中的"seconds"不符。故选 B。

45. A　题干:心肺复苏需要不间断地进行,直到专业医疗救助到达为止。文章最后一段表明,心肺复苏进行 15 次心脏按压,2 次人工呼吸,以此循环往复,直至专业医疗救助到达。故选 A。

Part Five

阅读和写作测试的第五部分是填词补文。这是一篇描述患者病情的报告,全文共十个空格,给出十二个词供选择。考生不仅要理解文章意思,而且要根据所提供单词的词性和词意选择符合上下文语境的词填入相应的空格。

46. H　本题考查"入院"的短语"be admitted to the hospital"。故选 H。

47. D　本题根据空格后面的症状"右腿和背部疼痛"。根据 of,在备选的词中,只有 complain 后面可以搭配 of/about,形成 complain of/about,中文意思是"主诉"。故选 D。

48. L　本题根据前文"疼痛八周前开始,在过去的几周内变得越发……",描述疼痛可以使用"severe"。故选 L。

49. C　本题空格在"do his work"后面,填写描述工作的副词,选项中"properly"符合上下文"无法正常工作"的意思。故选 C。

50. A　本题上下文表达"疼痛在夜间将患者痛醒"。根据"up"和备选词,可以推测"wake somebody up"。故选 A。

51. G　本题表达患者"右腿有刺痛感",使用介词"in"。故选 G。

52. E　本题上下文表达"体重减轻,约三公斤"。根据"lose"和"about three kilos",可选择"weight"。故选 E。

53. I　本题表达"患者因为疼痛加重而感到沮丧"。选项中表达情绪的词有"depressed"。故选 I。

54. J　本题表达"患者在检查后,被发现右脚脚趾麻木"。故选 J。

55. F　本题根据上下文表达"健康问题"。故选 F。

Part Six

56.

Attention to Avoiding Falling or Injury after a Stroke

If you suffer from stroke, you should clear the ways to the kitchen, bedroom and bathroom to keep you from being tripped up by any furniture. You are expected to wear comfortable shoes, keep the floor dry and use your walking frame even if it is a short distance. You should not walk in the dark and keep the bathroom light on at night. You'd better take your time when walking to avoid falling or injury.

Hopefully, you will keep the above tips in mind and provide a safe living environment for you and your family members at home.

Community Health Club

【审题】

阅读和写作测试的第六部分是写作。本题要求考生书写一则告示,宣传中风后如何防止摔倒。要求考生理解写作要求,读懂题目和提供的建议,使用完整并符合逻辑的句子写作。开始写作前,建议考生给自己的 Poster 一个 English title。除此之外,考生应根据本题提供的信息,确定合适的时态和语态。作文字数应在 80 个词左右。

【范文评述】

根据大纲的评分标准,从内容、结构和语言三方面对作文进行评析。文章标题醒目,使读者一目了然海报宣传的内容,能够将各条建议放在情境中表达,较单纯地陈述建议更为生动。所有建议信息没有遗漏,内容完整,语义符合逻辑。文章结构分为两部分,提出建议和表达希望的结束语,并附有告示的出处。全文词汇表达准确,使用了 trip up(绊倒),keep the bedroom light on at night 等较丰富的词汇,使语句具有画面感。语句时态语态一致,人称一致,无语言错误。

医护英语水平考试(一级)
模拟训练(二)

听力文本

This is METS-1 listening test. There are four parts to the test, parts One, Two, Three, and Four. You will hear each part twice. Now, look at the instructions for Part One. You will hear five patients describing their pain. Decide where each patient has the pain. Write the appropriate letter A—H in each box. Mark the corresponding letter on your answer sheet. You will hear each conversation twice. Here is an example:

Nurse (Woman): What's brought you here, Tim?

Patient (Man): My wrist is throbbing since I fell in the street.

The answer is in the wrist, so write letter F in the box. Now we are ready to start.

Conversation 1

Nurse (Woman): How do you feel this morning, Mr. Green?

Patient (Man): Awful. I've got a terrible headache.

Conversation 2

Nurse (Woman): What brought you to the emergency room, Bill?

Patient (Man): I fell down the stairs and broke my hip.

Conversation 3

Nurse (Woman): Hello, Mr. White. Are you feeling better today?

Patient (Man): Not really, I'm afraid. My neck aches a lot, especially in the morning.

Conversation 4

Nurse (Woman): Can you tell me the size and location of your wound, Robert?

Patient (Man): Sure. It is in the upper part of my back.

Conversation 5

Nurse (Man): Morning, Kathy. I'm here to do your dressing.

Patient (Woman): Thank you, Angela. I'll put my leg up for you.

This is the end of Part One. Now look at Part Two. You will hear a conversation of a nurse talking to a patient. For each of the following sentences, decide whether it is True (A) or False (B). Put a tick (√) in the relevant box. Mark the corresponding letter on your answer sheet. You will hear the conversation twice.

Nurse (Man): Good morning, this is Patient Registration Department. Have you been here before?

Patient (Woman): No. This is my first visit.

Nurse (Man): In this case, I have to ask you some questions. Can you tell me your full name, please?

Patient (Woman): Of course. My name is Jennifer Cotton.

Nurse (Man): OK. What's your date of birth, please?

Patient (Woman): The 28th of March, 1958.

Nurse (Man): 28th of March, 1958. Are you married or single?

Patient (Woman): I'm married.

Nurse (Man): One more question. Do you have any allergies?

Patient (Woman): Yes, I do. I'm allergic to peanuts.

Nurse (Man): OK. Now your hospital number is 6—8—1—5—4—9.

Patient (Woman): 6—8—1—5—4—9. Thank you.

Nurse (Man): You are welcome.

This is the end of Part Two. Now look at Part Three. You will hear a monologue of a nurse. For each of the following questions (or unfinished sentences), choose the correct answer A, B or C. Put a tick (√) in the relevant box. Mark the corresponding letter on your answer sheet. You will hear the monologue twice.

Nurse (Man): I work as an agency nurse and I specialize in renal care. This month I am working in a transplant unit, where I'm responsible for pediatric patients. I'm looking after a little girl who is waiting for a kidney transplant. I spend a lot of time with her, talking to her and explaining her condition. I carry out her tests and administer her medication every day, but we also play games. This week I'm teaching here to play dominos. I like communicating with my patients and don't like dealing with the paper work. Dealing with children can sometimes be very stressful, but it can also be very rewarding, too. I hope to qualify myself as an advanced practice nurse. In my free time, I go climbing, so you can find me in the mountains.

This is the end of Part Three. Now look at Part Four. You will hear a conversation of a nurse getting personal details from a patient. Fill in the blanks. Write the answers on your answer sheet. You will hear the conversation twice.

Nurse (Woman): Good morning. Mr. Bennett. I'm here to do your admission Obs.

Stephen (Man): Obs?

Nurse (Woman): Observations. It's your weight, temperature, pulse and respirations. Also your blood pressure and oxygen sats—that's the amount of oxygen in your blood.

Stephen (Man): Oh, right.

Nurse (Woman): First, I need to check your personal details. Can you tell me your full name, please?

Stephen (Man): Stephen Bennett.

Nurse (Woman): S-T-E-P-H-E-N. Stephen, Right?

Stephen (Man): Yes.

Nurse (Woman): What's your date of birth?

Stephen (Man): The 5th of May, 1980.

Nurse (Woman): OK. Now please stand on the scale.

Stephen (Man): Sure.

Nurse (Woman): Let me see. It's 75 kilos. Next, I'm going to take your temperature. I will take it in your ear with the tympanic thermometer.

Stephen (Man): Is that new?

Nurse (Woman): Yes. Your temperature is thirty-seven point two degrees centigrade.

Stephen (Man): That's all right.

Nurse (Woman): Yes. Now I will put the blood pressure cuff on. Can you roll up your sleeve, please?

Stephen (Man): No problem.

Nurse (Woman): This machine can read your blood pressure and pulse.

Stephen (Man): Mm. How are my readings?

Nurse (Woman): Your BP's a hundred and twenty over seventy-eight. That's normal. Your pulse is 68. That's also fine.

Stephen (Man): How about my oxygen sats?

Nurse (Woman): I will clip the lead on to your finger. ... Mm, the oxygen sats are 98%. That's fine, too.

Stephen (Man): Great. Thank you.

This is the end of Part Four. You now have five minutes to write your answers on the answer sheet. You have one more minute. This is the end of the listening test.

参考答案及解析

Ⅰ Listening

Part One

听力测试第一部分是信息匹配题。此部分检测考生是否已经掌握人类身体部位的相关医学英语词汇。考生听取护士与患者之间的对话后，理解患者对受伤部位或疼痛部位的描述，并对患者姓名和他们的伤痛部位进行信息匹配。

1. E　本题中病人自述头部疼痛（headache），故选 E。

2. D　本题中病人自述从楼梯摔下来，伤到了臀部（hip），故选 D。

3. G　本题中病人自述脖子（neck）疼痛，特别是在早上，故选 G。

4. A　本题中病人自述疼痛部位是背部（back）上方，故选 A。

5. C　本题中护士来给病人敷料，病人说把腿（leg）抬高些以方便护士敷料，故选 C。

Part Two

听力测试第二部分是信息判断题。考生听完护士对患者入院情况的询问后，根据患者所描述的病情信息，考生对所给的信息进行分析、判断。此部分的信息量较大，因此考生应按照题目顺序，完成作答。

6. B　本题中病人的姓名是 Jennifer Cotton，而不是 Lucy Cotton，故选 B。

7. A　本题中病人陈述出生日期是 1958 年 3 月 28 日，故选 A。

8. A　本题中病人陈述自己的婚姻状况是已婚，故选 A。

9. B　本题中病人陈述自己对花生（peanuts）过敏，而不是任何 nuts（坚果），故选 B。

10. B　本题中护士告诉病人编号是 681549，不是 681459，故选 B。

Part Three

听力测试第三部分是对医护人员的采访片段。考生听完后，要根据题干给出的信息和已经听到的内容，选择正确的答案。在答题时，考生应该关注题干的重点信息。

11. A　听力原文中提到目前护士在移植病房工作，故选 A。

12. B　听力原文中提到护士在照顾一个小女孩，故选 B。

13. C　听力原文中提到护士不喜欢案头工作（paper work），故选 C。

14. A　听力原文中提到他希望将来能够成为一名高级执业护士，故选 A。

15. B　听力原文中提到他在空闲时喜欢去爬山，故选 B。

Part Four

听力第四部分是信息填空题。考生在听完护士和病人的对话后，将正确的信息填在表格中题号后的空格内，每个空格只能填一个词或数字。

16. Stephen　听力原文中有拼写。

17. 75　听力原文中提到病人的体重是 75 千克。

18. 37.2　听力原文中提到病人的体温是 thirty-seven point two degrees centigrade。

19. Pulse　听力原文中提到脉搏是 68，故填 Pulse。

20. Oxygen sats　听力原文中提到氧饱和度（oxygen sats）是 98%。

II Reading and Writing

Part One

阅读和写作测试的第一部分是医院中常见物品、器械和基本的诊疗技术名称与其定义的匹配。此部分主要考查考生是否掌握了常见的医疗物品或器械的英语词汇。要求考生作答时,理解每一条定义和每一个物品或器械的名称,并进行匹配。

21. G 本句中描述的是用来注射或吸出液体的医疗用品,"syringe"指注射器,故选 G。

22. C 本句中描述的是通过拍摄骨骼图像进行检查,根据常识是 X 线检查,故选 C。

23. E 本句中描述的是能清晰显现血管的特殊染色剂,故选 E。

24. H 本句中描述用来帮助病人在病床上移动的装备,"hand block"指病床辅助手柄,故选 H。

25. D 本句中描述的是一种用来缓解肌肉酸痛的热垫,故选 D。

Part Two

第二部分是信息匹配,考查考生理解常见医护环境中简短信息的能力。要求考生将 5 句陈述与所给出的 7 个选项中的 5 个选项相匹配。答题时,考生应从标识或标签中寻找到与题干描述相符的关键词。考生应先明确左侧陈述的意思,从右侧信息中筛选。

26. E 本题干表示你要通过医生的处方来获取该药,说明此药是处方药,故选 E。

27. C 本题干表示点击此处找工作,C 选项显示的是个医疗就业网站,故选 C。

28. A 本题干描述的是病人在此候诊,故选 A。

29. D 本题干提示在服用该药时不能吃辛辣食物和海鲜。选项 D 中"restrain"和"avoid"表示克制和避免的意思,故选 D。

30. B 本题干提示该食物适合糖尿病人。糖尿病人应少吃或避免摄入糖分,选项 B "sugar-free"指无糖的,"recommend"指推荐,故选 B。

Part Three

第三部分是补全对话,考查考生理解常见医护环境中会话文本的能力。要求考生在通读全文的基础上,根据上下文从 8 个选项中选出 5 个最佳选项。答题时,考生需要仔细地将每个选项看完,根据上下文内容,针对每个情境去选择合适的应答句。

31. E 对话中上文护士要求病人要低盐饮食,下文中又说明因为病人有高血压,盐会引发高血压。由此推断,本句应是病人问护士为什么要低盐饮食,故选择 E。

32. C 对话中上文说到太多盐会引发高血压,所以护士要求病人低盐饮食,下文中护士给出了肯定赞许的回答"That's good",再分析所给选项意思,C 选项"我会在食物里少加些盐"应该是病人会说的话,故选 C。

33. A 对话中上文护士给病人一个不能吃的食物参照表,和下文中"yes"的肯定回答,结合选项,病人看完参照表后,表示过去不知道蒜盐里含盐是比较合理的选项,故选 A。

34. G 对话中下文护士回答冷冻蔬菜是可以吃的,推断出该句应是病人询问冷冻蔬菜可否吃,故选 G。

35. D 对话中下文"you are welcome"的回答可推断上文是表示感谢,故选 D。

Part Four

第四部分是信息判断题,考查考生通过理解常见医护短文获取重要信息的能力。要求考生在读懂全文的基础上,对给出的 10 个句子所表达的信息做出判断,从"正确""错误"或"未提及"三个选项中选出一个。本文是一篇有关焦虑的文章。

36. A 本题干说在危险时,焦虑会被激发出来。在文章的第一段提到焦虑是人们遇到危险或威胁时激发出来的身体报警系统,故选 A。

37. A 本题干说焦虑是一种重要的反应,它可能在紧急时刻拯救你的性命。在文章第一段说到"it serves an important basic survival function"它起到重要的基本生存作用,故选 A。

38. C 本题干中提到紧张时会感到眩晕"dizzy",但文章中没有提及,故选 C。

39. B 本题干说所有逃避反应就是呼吸、心跳加快、肌肉紧张,手心出汗……而在文章第二段说到这些反应只是逃避反应的一部分"part of the body's fight-flight response",而不是全部,故选 B。

40. C 本题干中说荷尔蒙也能引起逃避反应,但本文并未提及荷尔蒙,故选 C。

41. B 本题干说逃避反应在几秒钟内对所处环境做出判断,但文章第三段中说是由大脑做出判断的,故选 B。

42. A 本题干说当大脑解除所有紧张信号,我们就会放松下来。文章第三段最后一句话表达了相同的意思,故选 A。

43. B 本题干说焦虑引发的身体反应总是非常的激烈。在文章第二段最后一句话提到,这些反应有时温和,有时激烈,故选 B。

44. C 本题干意为如果你长时间保持警惕,你就会感到疲劳,而不再紧张焦虑。文章中没有提及,故选 C。

45. B 本题干说因为焦虑会起到重要的生存作用,所以我们需要越多焦虑越好。根据常识判断肯定是错误的,故选 B。

Part Five

第五部分是填词补文,通过词汇考查考生理解文章的能力。答题时,考生应该注意文中的时态、词的单复数、从句引导词、词组搭配、介词搭配等语法问题;兼顾语篇关系,前后参照,上下贯通。

46. E "BMI"指评估体重与身高比例的参考指数。本句中已有体重,所以选择"height"(身高)。

47. I 身体质量指数是用你的身高和体重来估计你身体的脂肪量,所以选择 I。

48. A "mark"可表示标示、标注。根据上下文可以判断出是要把测出的数值在图表上标示出来从而进行对比,故选择 A。

49. G 根据"percentiles""like"可以推断这个词应该和 percentiles 有相似的意思,再结合选项中的词汇,判断出选择 G。

50. K compare with 表示做比较,是固定搭配,故选择 K。

51. B 根据上文的"age",结合常识,这种对比应该是在相同年龄和性别的人群中比较才有意义,所以选择"gender"性别。

52. C "based on"基于、根据的意思。本句意思是根据图上的数值来判断你的身体质量指数是偏轻、正常、超重或是肥胖。

53. L 根据下面所列的词"healthy weight"健康体重,"overweight"超重,可以判断出这里应该是填体重过轻"underweight"。

54. D 同上题,这里可以判断出是肥胖"obese",故选 D。

55. F 根据本段的表达,这里应该是指到达 85 百分位数或者超过的(但是又不高于 95 百分位数)属于超重范畴,故选择 F。

Part Six

56.

A Case Report

John Green was admitted to Alexandra Hospital on August 26，2014 because he fell down the stairs and broke his hip. He was born on May 10，1995. He is single and studies in a college. His next of kin is his father，William，who can be contacted on 03762 - 578921. John is allergic to nothing. He has the family history of heart disease on his mother's side. He neither smokes nor drinks.

【审题】

读写第六部分是写作题。本题要求考生根据病历写一份报告。病历中提供的信息很详细,包括了病人的姓名、年龄、职业、婚姻状况、联系方式、生活习惯、入院原因、家族史及过敏史等内容。写作时要将这些信息用完整的句子表达出来,注意不要遗漏任何信息,正确使用标点符号,并将病历中出现的缩写用完整形式表达。此外,还应注意句子结构的完整性,可以结合信息使用恰当的连词,从而使文章内容更有逻辑性,字数应控制在 80 字以内。

【范文评述】

根据大纲的作文评分标准,从内容、结构和语言三方面对作文进行评析。在内容方面,文章对表格中所有信息进行了详细的转述,内容完整,无遗漏。在结构方面,句子衔接恰当,语意连贯。在语言方面,范文的语法结构使用准确,词汇运用恰当,文中使用了定语从句,把每个小信息有逻辑性地串联起来,使得文章内容全面且言简意赅。

医护英语水平考试(一级)

模拟训练(三)

听力文本

This is METS-1 listening test. There are four parts to the test，parts One，Two，Three，and Four. You will hear each part twice. Now，look at the instructions for Part One. You will hear five patients describing their pain. Decide where each patient has the pain. Write the appropriate letter A—H in each box. Mark the corresponding letter on your answer sheet. You will hear each conversation twice.

Here is an example:

Nurse (Woman): What's brought you here, Tim?
Patient (Man): My wrist is throbbing since I fell in the street.

The answer is in the wrist, so write letter F in the box. Now we are ready to start.

Conversation 1

Nurse (Man): Have you taken anything for the headache, Nancy?
Patient (Woman): Yes. I took some tablets, but they didn't work.

Conversation 2

Nurse (Man): Good morning, Lena. How are you today?
Patient (Woman): Now my nose is stuffed up and I have a sore throat.

Conversation 3

Nurse (Woman): What seems to be wrong, Richard?
Patient (Man): I've got an upset stomach. It's pretty bad.

Conversation 4

Nurse (Woman): What's your problem, Daniel?
Patient (Man): Well, I was hit by a car and when I got up, I had a sharp pain in my rib.

Conversation 5

Nurse (Woman): Is there anything I can do for you, Eason?
Patient (Man): Well, I've got the pain up and down my leg.

This is the end of Part One. Now look at Part Two. You will hear a conversation of a nurse talking to a patient. For each of the following sentences, decide whether it is True (A) or False (B). Put a tick (✓) in the relevant box. Mark the corresponding letter on your answer sheet. You will hear the conversation twice.

Nurse (Woman): Good morning, Ivan. I'm Judy, your charge nurse. How are you feeling today?
Patient (Man): I'm feeling much better than yesterday.
Nurse (Woman): Glad to hear that. Have you finished your breakfast?
Patient (Man): Yes, I have just had some bread.
Nurse (Woman): OK. May I give your tablet now?
Patient (Man): All right. What's it for?

15

Nurse (Woman): It's for lowering your blood pressure. Here you are. Take it immediatcly after meals.

Patient (Man): By the way, Dr. Biber has mentioned some antibiotics. Should I take now?

Nurse (Woman): According to the prescription, you should take them tomorrow.

Patient (Man): Should I take the antibiotics with meals?

Nurse (Woman): You can take them either with meals or on an empty stomach.

Patient (Man): I see. Thank you very much.

Nurse (Woman): You are welcome.

This is the end of Part Two. Now look at Part Three. You will hear a nurse explaining the admission procedure to a patient. For each of the following questions (or unfinished sentences), choose the correct answer A, B or C. Put a tick (✓) in the relevant box. Mark the corresponding letter on your answer sheet. You will hear the explanation twice.

Nurse (Woman): Good morning, my name is Cathy. Now I'd like to go through the admission procedure with you. First, you need to show your admission notice from your doctor. Then you can go to the payment hall to pay the advance deposit with your identity card. Usually, you will pay 5,000 *yuan* in advance, either in cash or by your card. And the payment hall is on the first floor. You can take the elevator to go downstairs over there. Then please come back to the nurse station with all the receipts you have, and I will arrange a ward for you. As the doctor has ordered a CT-scan of your abdomen, you may wait in your ward at 8 o'clock tomorrow morning, and the nurse will take you to the examination room. Remember not to eat or drink anything after midnight. The result will be ready the following day.

This is the end of Part Three. Now look at Part Four. You will hear a patient calling to make an appointment. Fill in the blanks. Write the answers on your answer sheet. You will hear the conversation twice.

Nurse (Woman): Hello, this is Saint Louis Hospital.

Justin (Man): Hello, can I make an appointment?

Nurse (Woman): Sure. What's your name?

Justin (Man): Justin Simpson.

Nurse (Woman): OK. Mr. Simpson, and your date of birth?

Justin (Man): April 16th, 1987.

Nurse (Woman): Have you ever been a patient at our hospital before?

Justin（Man）：No，this is my first time to make an appointment.

Nurse（Woman）：Would you please tell me your insurance card number?

Justin（Man）：375642.

Nurse（Woman）：OK. Which department do you want to register with?

Justin（Man）：Department of Medicine，I guess. I want to see a physician.

Nurse（Woman）：What's wrong with you?

Justin（Man）：Recently，I've got a pain in my chest and it makes me uncomfortable. I think I need to have a check.

Nurse（Woman）：Which doctor do you want to visit?

Justin（Man）：Dr. Smith. Does he provide outpatient service this week?

Nurse（Woman）：Yeah，the available time will be 8 o'clock Tuesday morning，2 o'clock Wednesday afternoon，and 1 o'clock Thursday afternoon. What time is convenient for you?

Justin（Man）：I think I would be fine on Wednesday afternoon.

Nurse（Woman）：That's fine，but there're other three patients before you. Do you mind waiting for about an hour?

Justin（Man）：No.

Nurse（Woman）：Well，let me make your appointment at 3 o'clock Wednesday afternoon with Dr. Smith.

Justin（Man）：OK，thank you very much.

Nurse（Woman）：You are welcome. Bye.

Justin（Man）：Bye.

This is the end of Part Four. You now have four minutes to write your answers on the answer sheet. You have one more minute. This is the end of the listening test.

参考答案及解析

I Listening

Part One

1. A 本题中护士询问病人头痛服药情况（headache）。

2. B 本题中病人自述喉咙疼痛（sore throat）。

3. D 本题中病人自述胃部不适（upset stomach）。

4. E 本题中病人提及被车撞倒，起来后肋骨（rib）剧痛。

5. G 本题中病人自述腿部（leg）疼痛。

Part Two

6. B 本题中病人自述感觉比昨天好很多。

7. A 本题中病人回答已吃过一些面包当早餐。

8. A　本题中护士回答病人所服药片的作用为降血压。

9. B　本题中病人询问护士医生所开的抗生素是否需要今天服用时，护士回答根据处方单显示，明天才需要服用。

10. B　本题中护士指出医生所开的抗生素既可随餐服用也可以空腹服用。

Part Three

11. A　听力原文中提到办理入院手续需要携带入院通知和身份证。

12. C　听力原文中提到预付金既可以用现金，也可以刷卡。

13. B　听力原文中提到入院后，会安排病人进行腹部CT扫描。

14. B　听力原文中提到将由护士带领病人去检查室。

15. C　听力原文中提到检查结果将在第二天获得。

Part Four

16. Male　护士称呼患者为Mr. Simpson，表明了患者的性别。

17. 375642　护士询问患者保险卡的号码，病人直接回答了卡号。

18. Medicine　听力原文中提到病人因胸部不适，要求挂号内科（Department of Medicine），找内科医生（physician）检查。

19. chest　听力原文中提到病人胸部疼痛。

20. three　听力原文中提到医生星期三下午两点有空，但前面已安排其他三位病人，病人同意等待一小时。

II　Reading and Writing

Part One

21. F　用于涂在肌肤或伤口上帮助恢复的光滑物质是药膏（ointment）。

22. E　用于检查或记录身体运行过程的器械为监护仪（monitor）。

23. B　用于拍摄人体内部器官图片的技术即为超声波（ultrasound）。

24. C　用于接送病人出入医院的交通工具是救护车（ambulance）。

25. H　内含粉状或液体状药品，可吞咽的细小管状物品是胶囊（capsule）。

Part Two

26. E　题干描述的"不需付钱"，与选项"免费（free of charge）"的意思一致。

27. C　题干中"surgery"与选项中"operation"意思一致，都有"手术"之意。

28. D　题干描述患者为两岁男童，与选项中四个月以上婴幼儿用药指导的年龄范围一致。

29. A　题干描述紧急情况下提供帮助，A选项是求助热线号码，符合题干要求。

30. B　题干提及阅读相关材料，与选项B"Guidebook"范围相符。

Part Three

31. D　根据病人回答"约一个月"，推断出护士就患病时间进行提问，与D选项中"How long"提问范围符合。

32. C　对话中病人提及服用过安眠药，但不起作用，与C选项中是否服用过药物问题相一致。

33. A　对话中护士提出是否有头疼的问题，A项不仅回答"有时候"（sometimes），还列举出其他相关症状"胃口不好"(a poor appetite)和"易于紧张"(stressed)。

34. G 对话中病人询问解决办法,与 G 选项中的多休息(more rest),不要过于紧张(don't strain yourself)的回答相符。

35. F 对话中出现"Thank you very much",可推断出下文是表示不用谢"You are welcome"。

Part Four

36. B 题干意思是"糖尿病仅发生在成年人身上",与文章第一段第一句"成人与儿童都会患糖尿病"的论述相悖。

37. B 题干意思是"糖尿病患者细胞将吸收更多葡萄糖",与文章第一段中"因体内缺少胰岛素或细胞对胰岛素有排异,糖尿病患者细胞内缺乏葡萄糖"论述不一致。

38. C 题干意思是"糖尿病分为 1 型和 2 型",文章中未提及。

39. A 题干意思是"影响体内葡萄糖的成分是胰岛素",与文章中第一段陈述内容相符。

40. C 题干意思是"糖尿病是世界上最常见疾病之一",文章未涉及此方面内容。

41. A 题干意思是"糖尿病人总往厕所跑",与文章第二段最后一句意思相同。

42. B 题干意思是"细胞吸收葡萄糖后,还会寻找替代物并最终吸收肌肉的能量",这与文章第三段第二句"因未能吸收足够葡萄糖,细胞吸收肌肉能量,使糖尿病患者体重剧降"的意思相悖。

43. A 题干意思是"如果你感到不明原因的虚弱和疲倦,你可能患上糖尿病",与文章第四段第一句"糖尿病的另一预兆是会感到不明原因的虚弱和疲倦"的意思相符。

44. B 题干意思是"一些糖尿病患者更容易显胖",与第三段中糖尿病患者会急剧消瘦的论述不符。

45. C 题干意思是"人们已经发明许多新药来治疗糖尿病",此观点在文章中没有出现。

Part Five

46. I 文章首句指出 diet 这个词汇到处出现,后面列举出 diet Coke,diet Pepsi,diet pills,on-fat diet,vegetable diet 等例子,同时该单词首字母需要大写,确定为"Examples"。

47. D 本题考查被动语态用法,需要选择动词的过去分词形式,本句词组为 be attracted by,意为"被……所吸引"。

48. J 动词 stop 后接动词-ing 形式,且这个-ing 形式的动词后面可接介词 about。

49. A 此空格为减肥食品带来的积极或消极影响,故在选项 A 和 G 中选择。根据前文内容,作者对减肥食品持否定态度。

50. E Not only … ,but also … 的用法应前后保持一致,词组 lie in 结构中的介词 in 不能省。

51. H 本题考查副词的用法。此空格需要一个副词来修饰形容词 dangerous,选项中只有"potentially"一个副词,意为"潜在地"。

52. K 本题考查固定搭配。"be aware of"意为"意识到"。

53. F 英语中句子的连接要用连词,选项中仅有的连词"once",意思为"一旦"。

54. B 作者一直对减肥食品持否定态度,呼吁大家进行抵制(resist)。

55. C　根据上下文,减肥食品无论从心理(psychological)上还是在生理(physical)上,都给人们带来了伤害。前面已经提到心理危害。

Part Six

56.

A Case Report

The patient Nora Hanks, female, 42-year-old, was hospitalized on July 18th, 2014. She complained of having a headache and vomiting in the morning. Her respiratory rate was 38 per minute and pulse rate was 130 per minute. Her temperature was recorded as 37.5 ℃ and her blood pressure was 180/140 mmHg. She was diagnosed with hypertension (high blood pressure). According to the doctor's order, she had been given some anti-hypertensive drugs and she started to have a low-salt diet. No further complication was noted so far.

【审题】

写作部分要求考生根据入院单写一份报告。入院单中提供的信息很详细,包括了病人的姓名、年龄、性别、入院时间、入院原因、生命体征及护理过程等内容,写作时应将这些信息尽量表达完整,无遗漏。表格中出现的缩写用完整形式表达,字数应不少于 80 个词。

【范文评述】

根据大纲的作文评分标准,从内容、结构和语言三方面对作文进行评析。在内容方面,紧紧围绕"入院"这一主题,对入院单中所有信息进行了详细的转述,内容完整,无遗漏。在结构方面,句子衔接恰当,语意连贯。从介绍患者的基本信息到介绍入院时间及入院时的症状,然后叙述患者入院后各项生命体征、诊断结果、治疗措施,最后介绍患者目前的病情,这完全符合入院治疗程序,符合逻辑。医学英语属于科技英语的分支,具备自身独特的语言特点,要求语言客观、简练、准确,使用大量的专业术语和被动语态。所以,在语言方面,范文的语法结构使用准确,词汇运用恰当,文中使用了大量医学术语,如 vomit,respiratory rate,pulse,hypertension 等;被动语态包括 be hospitalized,be diagnosed with,be given anti-hypertensive drugs 等。

医护英语水平考试(一级)

模拟训练(四)

听力文本

This is METS-1 listening test. There are four parts in the test, parts One, Two, Three, and Four. You will hear each part twice. Now, look at the instructions for Part One. You will hear five patients describing their pain. Decide where each patient has the pain. Write the appropriate letter A—H in each box. Mark the corresponding letter on your answer sheet. You will hear each conversation twice.

Here is an example：

Nurse（Woman）：What's brought you here, Tim?
Patient（Man）：My wrist has been throbbing since I fell in the street.

The answer is in the wrist, so write letter F in the box. Now we are ready to start.

Conversation 1

Nurse（Woman）：Hello, Sam. How are you feeling today?
Patient（Man）：My chest still hurts from time to time.

Conversation 2

Nurse（Man）：Do you have any discomfort, Judy?
Patient（Woman）：Yes. My ankle aches a lot.

Conversation 3

Nurse（Woman）：What's wrong with you, Bill?
Patient（Man）：I fell off the stairs this morning and hurt my knees.

Conversation 4

Nurse（Woman）：Good morning, Martin. What's your problem?
Patient（Man）：My wisdom tooth has been bothering me.

Conversation 5

Nurse（Man）：How can I help you, Linda?
Patient（Woman）：Well, I have no idea. But I have a sharp stomachache.

This is the end of Part One. Now look at Part Two. You will hear a conversation between a nurse and a patient. For each of the following sentences, decide whether it is True（A）or False（B）. Put a tick（✓）in the relevant box. Mark the corresponding letter on your answer sheet. You will hear the conversation twice.

Nurse（Woman）：Good morning, Mr. Parsons.
Patient（Man）：Good morning.
Nurse（Woman）：It is time for you to go home. I have some tips for you.
Patient（Man）：Well, that must be helpful.
Nurse（Woman）：First of all, you cannot have too much salt in your food. Too much salt

21

is bad for your blood pressure.

Patient (Man): OK，I will do it. Anything else?

Nurse (Woman): Second，you need to stop drinking beer because it has a lot of calories. This is a book for you. If you are not sure about something，you can read it.

Patient (Man): Thanks. I'll read it then.

Nurse (Woman): How is your appetite? Do you feel like eating?

Patient (Man): No. I sometimes don't feel hungry. And the food is not tasty without salt.

Nurse (Woman): Yes，I can understand. The doctor says your blood pressure is stable now. You need to keep it.

Patient (Man): Oh，glad to hear that. Thank you very much.

This is the end of Part Two. Now look at Part Three. You will hear a monologue of a doctor talking about adult acne. For each of the following questions or unfinished sentences，choose the correct answer A，B or C. Put a tick (✓) in the relevant box. Mark the corresponding letter on your answer sheet. You will hear the monologue twice.

Doctor (Woman): There are a lot of reasons for adult acne. But mostly it is because of pressure and the endocrine disorder coming after that. Think about it. Are you living a regular life，like eating regularly or sleeping regularly? If you don't want to get acne，you have to keep a regular lifestyle. Here are some instructions for you. First of all，you should wash your face with warm water and mild soap three times a day. Washing will keep pores open and clear away extra oil. Second，don't touch your face with hands. Touching may cause very serious infection. Third，don't eat too much fat or spicy food such as onion or curry. Since you have got acne，you can use this cream. Put the cream onto your face twice a day，before going to bed at night and when you get up next morning. Remember to clean your face each time you use it.

This is the end of Part Three. Now look at Part Four. You will hear a conversation between a doctor and a patient. Fill in the blanks. Write the answers on your answer sheet. You will hear the conversation twice.

Doctor (Woman): Good morning. How can I help you?

Patient (Man): Good morning，doctor. I keep coughing, and it won't stop.

Doctor (Woman): OK. Now I will ask you several questions. Please answer my questions so I can fill in the record. What is your name?

Patient（Man）：My name is Tim Hiddleston. H-I-D-D-L-E-S-T-O-N，Hiddleston.

Doctor（Woman）：And your phone number?

Patient（Man）：It's 4225329682.

Doctor（Woman）：When did you begin to cough?

Patient（Man）：Last week.

Doctor（Woman）：Do you have a fever?

Patient（Man）：Yes. I took my temperature at home. It was 38 degrees celsius.

Doctor（Woman）：Do you have any other symptoms?

Patient（Man）：Yes, I have a chest pain sometimes.

Doctor（Woman）：How often is the pain? And what is it like?

Patient（Man）：It's a sharp pain on the right side of my chest.

Doctor（Woman）：You'd better have an ECG and X-ray examination to see if there is an infection.

Patient（Man）：All right. I hope there isn't any infection.

Doctor（Woman）：Of course. Are you allergic to any medicine or food?

Patient（Man）：Yes. I'm allergic to fish.

Doctor（Woman）：OK. That's all the information I need. And this is the X-ray examination list. You can take it with you to the X-ray room.

Patient（Man）：Thank you.

This is the end of Part Four. You now have five minutes to write your answers on the answer sheet. You have one more minute. This is the end of the listening test.

参考答案及解析

Ⅰ Listening

Part One

1. C 本题中患者自述胸痛,故选 C。

2. G 本题患者脚踝痛,故选 G。

3. D 患者自述摔下楼梯伤到膝盖,故选 D。

4. H 患者饱受智齿困扰,故选 H。

5. E 患者胃部剧痛,故选 E。

Part Two

6. A 对话开始护士便说患者即将出院,有一些事项需要注意,故本句正确。

7. A 根据对话,患者觉得食欲不振,原因是饮食减少了盐分摄入,故本句正确。

8. B 护士提醒患者不能喝啤酒,因为啤酒热量过高,没有说患者过胖。本句错误。

9. A 护士说患者血压现在已经稳定,故本句正确。

10. A 护士对患者的情况很了解,而且耐心讲解出院后需要注意的事项,因此可以说护士对患者非常耐心,故正确。

Part Three

11. A 患者长了粉刺,来看皮肤科医生,故选 A。

12. C 对话中说长粉刺的原因是压力大,以及内分泌失调,没提到抑郁,故选 C。

13. B 医生让患者用温水洗脸,故选 B。

14. A 医生的医嘱中提到辛辣食物会导致长粉刺,故选 A。

15. B 根据医嘱,药膏早晚各用一次,一天两次,故选 B。

Part Four

16. Hiddleston 根据患者回答的拼写来确定。

17. cough 患者的症状是咳嗽、胸痛以及高烧。

18. 38 患者自述在家量的体温是 38 摄氏度。

19. X-ray 医生检查后认为患者需要拍心电图及 X 光片。

20. fish 患者自述对鱼过敏。

Ⅱ Reading and Writing

Part One

21. G 用来量体温的工具是温度计,故选 G。

22. F 外科医生用手术刀做手术,故选 F。

23. B 医生用听诊器听病人的心跳和呼吸,故选 B。

24. D 核磁共振可用来检查人体内部组织,故选 D。

25. H 用来清理伤口的应该是棉签,故选 H。

Part Two

26. C 在医生指导下使用。

27. D 该处禁止吸烟。

28. A 患者血糖高,应选择无糖饮食 sugar-free diet。

29. E 该处是患者突发疾病时的去处,应该是急诊室 emergency room。

30. B 如非必要请远离此处,应该是有危险的地方,radiation risk 即辐射危害。

Part Three

31. E 本句下一行患者回答 No. This is the first time.“这是第一次”,所以问题应该是“你以前来过吗?”,即 Have you ever been here before?

32. B 下一行的回答是 Yes, I do,提问也应该是 Do 开头的疑问句。

33. G 上一行问题问“挂什么科看病”,空格后面说 My tooth aches badly. 患者牙疼,那么应该要看牙医。

34. C 后一句说 Please don't lose it and bring it whenever you come. 提醒不要弄丢某样东西,本处应该交付这件东西,即 C 项提到的 registration card,登记卡。

35. A 本空下一行的回答是指路,因此本空问路,因此选 A。

Part Four

36. A 根据文章第一段第三句 despite her youthful appearance 可知 Lily Cook 比实际年龄显年轻。

37. A 第二段第一句给出。

38. B 第二段第二句 Chronological age is determined by birthday.

39. B 第二段第三句提到 RealAge 是一家从事健康产业的公司。

40. A 第三段第一句。导致衰老的因素有很多,抽烟是其中一种。

41. B 第三段第一句。睡眠也会影响衰老,因此表述错误。

42. C 第三段第一句提到睡眠对衰老的影响,但是没有说缺乏睡眠会如何,因此选项未提及。

43. B 第三段第一句提到 The online test set by the company is free. 网上测试是免费的,因此表述错误。

44. A 第三段第二句提到 RealAge may request detailed personal health information from you. 该公司需要详细的个人健康信息做评估。

45. A 第三段第三句,... they will give you a personalized plan to help you feel younger ... ,公司会针对个人制定个性化方案。

Part Five

46. C 此处在 was 后,介词 to 前,考虑动词搭配 admit somebody to a place,安排某人入院。

47. E 本空填名词,他的"症状"变糟,即 symptom。

48. H 此空填动词过去时态,结合句意,前半句话说患者晚上病情严重,半夜会"醒来",即 woke。

49. L 本空所在句子结构完整,考虑填入副词完善句意,即填 gradually。

50. D 根据句子结构判断本处填动词过去时态,结合句意,疼痛随后"传播"到其他部位,即 spread。

51. F 本空填入名词和 and 前面的 position 并列,疼痛和患者的姿势以及"动作"有关,即 movement。

52. K 本空在句中做主语,应填入名词,X 光"检查"发现有胸腔积液,即 examination。

53. G 此处填入动词,用胸腔引流这种方法来"治疗",即 treat。

54. B 自从患病以来,患者没有明显的"体重"下降,即 weight。

55. J 本处需要填入一个词修饰 examination,考虑形容词,需要进行"进一步"检查,即 further。

Part Six

56.

A Case Report

Ms. Emma Roberts, born on February 14, 1984, was admitted to hospital on June 26, 2017. Her contact number is 37784005279. Upon admission, she had symptoms of headache and vomiting. According to the physical examinations, her temperature is 38 degrees centigrade, her pulse rate is 108 beats per minute, and her respiratory rate is 24 breaths per minute. Apart from those, her blood pressure is 120 over 80. An X-ray examination and a blood test are needed to establish an accurate diagnosis.

【审题】

这是一篇关于患者入院记录的写作。要求考生写不少于 80 个词,内容应包括病人姓名、年龄、联系方式、体格检查等。表格中的信息要尽量表述完整,无遗漏;但也要注意不要超词太多。考生应注意使用常见的表达用语,如 be admitted to hospital/be hospitalized。另需注意 T 代表体温,P 代表脉搏频率,R 代表呼吸频率,BP 代表血压。

【范文评述】

本篇范文内容翔实,涵盖试题提供的所有细节,包括病人姓名、年龄、联系方式、体格检查等。语言通顺,无病句或其他语法错误。时态使用方面十分妥帖,第一句用过去时陈述入院时间这一过去事实;后文使用一般现在时,因其内容为病人症状描述。语言使用上也有可圈可点之处,如介词短语 Upon admission 言简意赅地表达"患者刚入院的时候"这层意思。用并列句列举患者脉搏频率、呼吸频率、血压的分别数值,结构清楚明了。

医护英语水平考试(一级)

模拟训练(五)

听力文本

This is METS-1 listening test. There are four parts to the test, parts One, Two, Three, and Four. You will hear each part twice. Now, look at the instructions for Part One. You will hear five patients describing their pain. Decide where each patient has the pain. Write the appropriate letter A—H in each box. Mark the corresponding letter on your answer sheet. You will hear each conversation twice.

Here is an example:

Nurse (Woman): What brought you here, Tim?
Patient (Man): My wrist has been throbbing since I fell in the street.

The answer is in the wrist, so write letter F in the box. Now we are ready to start.

Conversation 1

Nurse (Woman): Good morning, Blake. Could you tell me what's wrong with you?
Patient (Man): I feel terrible. I have a really bad headache and a stiff neck.

Conversation 2

Nurse（Woman）：So，what happened to you，Paul?

Patient（Man）：I was injured in a car accident，and I had a sharp pain in my back.

Conversation 3

Nurse（Woman）：You look pale，Jack. What's the problem?

Patient（Man）：Well，my right knee hurts a lot and I can't sleep the whole night.

Conversation 4

Nurse（Woman）：Hello，Susan. How are you feeling today?

Patient（Man）：I've had a chest pain for a few days. My temperature keeps going up and down as well.

Conversation 5

Nurse（Woman）：What brought you here，Mike?

Patient（Man）：I feel very tired and have a sore throat. I have a running nose and I keep sneezing.

This is the end of Part One. Now look at Part Two. You will hear a conversation of a nurse talking to a patient. For each of the following sentences，decide whether it is True (A) or False (B). Put a tick (✓) in the relevant box. Mark the corresponding letter on your answer sheet. You will hear the conversation twice.

Dr. Hehn（Woman）：Good evening，Paul. Could I have a look at your hand?

Paul（Man）：Sure.

Dr. Hehn（Woman）：So，how did you cut your hand?

Paul（Man）：It was an accident at work. I am a builder and often work with a knife.

Dr. Hehn（Woman）：Oh，I see. That is why the wound is such a deep cut. But don't worry. Cuts with knives usually heal quickly. When did you last have a tetanus injection?

Paul（Man）：I have no idea. Maybe it was a long time ago，but I can't really remember.

Dr. Hehn（Woman）：Well，you'll need a tetanus injection，then.

Paul（Man）：All right.

Dr. Hehn（Woman）：And then I'm afraid it will need a couple of stitches.

Paul（Man）：I guess it needs stitches. That's why I come here.

Dr. Hehn（Woman）：Right，let's clean the wound first.

Paul（Man）：Oh，I am scared.

Dr. Hehn (Woman): Don't worry. You will recover soon.

This is the end of Part Two. Now look at Part Three. You will hear a conversation between a nurse and a patient. For each of the following questions (or unfinished sentences), choose the correct answer A, B or C. Put a tick (✓) in the relevant box. Mark the corresponding letter on your answer sheet. You will hear the conversation twice.

Nurse (Woman): Hello, Gary. How do you feel today?

Patient (Man): Hello, Eliza, I feel much better today. I've got a question. Is it true that fever is not a disease itself?

Nurse (Woman): Yes, it is true. Fever is a symptom of many diseases, such as pneumonia, some cancers, stroke or heart attack. Fever helps the body to fight against these diseases.

Patient (Man): What temperature would be harmful to our health?

Nurse (Woman): A fever of 39 ℃ or higher needs special care, and temperatures above 44.5 ℃ are usually fatal.

Patient (Man): Then how could a high temperature be brought down?

Nurse (Woman): In most cases, fever can be reduced by aspirin or other fever-reducing drugs. You can also sponge down a fever. Wring towels half-dry and sponge the forehead, face, ears, neck, body, armpits, groins, arms and legs.

Patient (Man): Should we eat as usual?

Nurse (Woman): Yes. If you have a poor appetite, just eat as much as you like. You should drink a lot of water, fruit juice, milk, or clear soup. Cold drinks can lower body temperature. If a fever persists for more than 5 days, you should go to seek medical treatment.

Patient (Man): Thank you very much.

This is the end of Part Three. Now look at Part Four. You will hear a conversation in the Outpatient Department between a nurse and a patient. Fill in the blanks. Write the answers on your answer sheet. You will hear the conversation twice.

Nurse (Woman): Sir, have you registered yet?

Patient (Man): No, I haven't.

Nurse (Woman): Are you a medical or surgical case?

Patient (Man): I am a medical case.

Nurse (Woman): Do you have your history sheet?

Patient (Man): Yes, here you are.

Nurse（Woman）：What's wrong with you?

Patient（Man）：I found blood in my urine. My blood pressure is 140/90. My pulse is 75 per minute and I sleep for about 8 hours every night.

Nurse（Woman）：Let me fill in this admission card. What's your name?

Patient（Man）：Wentworth Connolly.

Nurse（Woman）：Your marital status, age, profession?

Patient（Man）：I am married, 30 years old and I am an engineer.

Nurse（Woman）：Oh, let me see. Now your hospital number is 654321.

Patient（Man）：Thanks.

Nurse（Woman）：... So it is April 3 today, and you are admitted.

Patient（Man）：Thank you.

This is the end of Part Four. You now have five minutes to write your answers on the answer sheet. You have one more minute. This is the end of the listening test.

参考答案及解析

I Listening

Part One

1. D 本题中患者自述头痛(have a really bad headache)，故选 D。

2. H 本题中患者自述在事故中受伤，后背疼痛厉害(I had a sharp pain in my back)，故选 H。

3. A 本题中患者自述右膝盖受伤(My right knee hurts a lot)，故选 A。

4. B 本题中患者自述胸痛数日(I've had a chest pain)，体温忽高忽低，故选 B。

5. G 本题中患者自述喉咙疼痛(have a sore throat)，打喷嚏，流鼻涕，故选 G。

Part Two

6. A 患者说他是一名建筑工人，平时工作使用刀，本句正确。

7. B 根据对话，患者的刀伤很深，故本句错误。

8. B 根据对话，医生告诉患者刀伤很容易愈合，本句错误。

9. A 医生告诉患者他需要进行破伤风注射，本句正确。

10. A 患者告诉医生他之所以来看医生，是因为他觉得他的伤口应该缝合，故正确。

Part Three

11. C 根据短文内容，发热可以帮助肌体战胜疾病，提高抵抗力，故选 C。

12. C 根据短文内容，发热 39 ℃或者更高一些就需要特别注意；如果发热温度超过 44.5 ℃就致命了(Temperatures above 44.5 ℃ are usually fatal.)，故选 C。

13. A 根据短文内容，可以采用服用阿司匹林等退烧药来缓解发热症状，故选 A。

14. B 根据短文内容，如果持续发热 5 天以上，必须去看医生，故选 B。

15. B 根据短文内容，发热还可以通过喝冷饮来降温，故选 B。

Part Four

16. April 3　根据护士的描述确定患者的入院日期。

17. Married　患者告诉医生他已婚。

18. Engineer/An engineer　根据患者的回答来确定。

19. Blood　根据患者自述确定答案(I found blood in my urine)。

20. 140/90　根据患者自述确定答案。

Ⅱ　Reading and Writing

Part One

21. G　ICU 是 Intensive Care Unit"重症监护室"的缩写,专门收治危重患者。

22. F　本题所述设备是用来测量体重的,scale 解释为"刻度"或者"秤",故选 F。

23. B　用于拍摄人体内部器官图片的技术是超声波(ultrasound),故选 B。

24. D　注射器 syringe 是一种常见的医疗用具,主要用以注射药液或抽液,故选 D。

25. H　elbow 是上臂与前臂之间的关节或胳膊弯曲处,故选 H。

Part Two

26. B　该选项标识的内容是"避免暴露在阳光下",符合题干的描述。

27. F　该选项标识的内容是"残疾人专用坡道",符合题干的描述。

28. E　该选项标识的内容是"用氧　此处禁止吸烟",符合题干的描述。

29. A　该选项标识的内容是"危险! 医疗废弃物",符合题干的描述。

30. D　该选项标识的内容是"此处为医院候诊区",符合题干的描述。

Part Three

31. C　通过医生的问话 How long have you had this problem? 推断第一句中患者在诉说自己的症状。选项 C 中患者描述自己的失眠症状,符合上下题意,故选 C。

32. F　对话中上文医生问患者有这个症状多久了(How long have you had this problem?),患者回答三个月,符合上下文题意,故选 F。

33. A　对话中上文医生问患者有没有服过药(Have you taken any medicine?),患者回答服过安眠药(sleeping pills),符合上下文,故选 A。

34. D　医生给患者测量血压,然后给出的判断是患者因工作劳累(You are just a little exhausted from overwork.)导致前面提到的失眠症状,根据题意,故选 D。

35. B　患者询问医生应该怎么办(What should I do then?),医生给出建议 I think you need more rest. Don't strain yourself too much(我认为你需要多休息,不要太辛苦)符合上下文,故选 B。

Part Four

36. B　原文第二段第一句得知:There is no cure for AIDS or no vaccine to prevent it. 艾滋病无法治愈也没有疫苗可以预防。

37. A　原文第二段第四句 The virus invades healthy cells including white blood cells that are part of our defense system against disease. 题干句子是此句的一个同义替换,意思为"当病毒入侵我们的免疫系统时,也开始破坏我们的白细胞"。

38. B　原文第二段第七句 And the viral particles move on to invade and kill more

healthy cells(病毒颗粒继续入侵并杀死更多的健康细胞)来判断,题干意思与原句相反。

39. C 虽然根据常识可以判断,苍蝇不会传播艾滋病,但是原文中并没有提及。

40. A 原文第三段第一句 The AIDS virus is carried in a person's body fluids. 可以推断人的体液中携带艾滋病毒。

41. B 原文第三段第三句 It also can be passed in blood products or from a pregnant woman with AIDS to her developing baby. (艾滋病毒可以通过血液制品和母婴传播。)如果孕妇携带艾滋病毒,婴儿也会感染艾滋病毒。

42. B 原文第四段末句 Experts say no one has gotten AIDS by living with, caring for or touching an AIDS patient. 可以推断,握手是 touching 的一种,是不会感染艾滋病毒的。

43. B 原文第四段末句 Experts say no one has gotten AIDS by living with, caring for or touching an AIDS patient. 可以推断,照顾艾滋病人是不会被传染艾滋病的。

44. C 原文末段第一句 There are several warning signs of an AIDS infection. They include ... 并没有提及剧烈的头疼是感染艾滋病毒的症状或征兆。

45. A 根据原文末段的第一句 There are several warning signs of an AIDS infection. They include ... 可以推断接下来描述的是艾滋病的一些症状。

Part Five

46. H 根据原文中的 one of ... 判断,此处需要一个名词,且是一个复数名词。选项中只有 H symptoms 是复数名词,意思为症状。

47. C 根据所在句子结构来判断,此处需要一个定语从句的连接词,先行词是前面的 men 和 women。此空格可推断为可以指代"人"的连接代词且在定语从句中做主语。选项 C who 符合语法和句意。

48. A 此处需要一个动词,空格的前面是情态动词 can。由此推断应填一个动词原形,符合此要求的有 affect 和 do,由于空格的后面是宾语 non-smokers,排除了动词 do,故选 A。

49. L 本句的意思是被诊断为肺癌的妇女中,20%从来都没有吸过烟,诊断 diagnose 这个词与介词 with 是固定搭配,因此 L 从词义及动词形式均符合要求。

50. B 选项后面是动词原形 have,说明此空格可能是一个副词,或情态动词,或表示强调的助动词 do 或 does(由主语单复数决定)。备选项中没有副词和情态动词,所以 B 选项符合语法要求。

51. G lung cancer 是文中作者讨论的中心话题,因此要选 G 项的 lung 与 cancer 搭配。

52. D be sure 后面引导一个宾语从句,符合要求的是 D 选项 why 和 C 选项 who,根据所在句子的意思,医生不能确定为什么不吸烟的年轻妇女也会患肺癌,why 在定语从句中做原因状语,who 是代词,不能做状语。故 D 选项符合要求。

53. F It could be 和宾语 factors 之间需要一个介词引出一个逻辑关系,因为 factors 的前面已经有了修饰词 environmental,所以就不再考虑选择形容词,再根据上下文句意,故推断出选择介词短语 due to(由于),选项 F 正确。

54. J 此句意思十分明确,此空格应填与厨房相关的词,选项 cooking 符合句意,"所释放的难闻的气味来自厨房的油烟",因此选 J。

55. K 本题考查的是固定搭配 tend to,意思为"倾向于……,易于……",所以选 K。

Part Six

56.

A Case Report

Mr. Robert Naton is a 51-year-old male patient. He is married and now he works as a bus driver. His next of kin is his daughter, Susan, and his contact number is 4665 048 5726. Mr. Robert Naton was admitted to hospital because of heart disease. He has had heart disease for about seven years. He has a family history of heart disease on his father's side. The patient doesn't smoke or drink. He is allergic to seafood.

【审题】

本题要求根据病历书写报告,病历中提供了非常详细的患者信息,包括患者的姓名、年龄、性别、职业、婚姻状况、生活习惯、联系方式、家族史和过敏史等方面的内容。因此,在写作时只需要将这些信息用句子的形式完整地表达出来即可。注意:不可遗漏任何信息,标点符号要正确使用。时态的选择也是不可忽视的。根据病历内容,患者信息是作文的主要内容,因此,本文时态应以一般现在时态为主。此外,还要清楚病例中的字母缩写表达的含义,在写作时要用完整的表达形式进行描述。写作时还要注意句子结构的完整性及句子之间的逻辑性,适当使用承转启合的连接词,并且文章的字数也应符合要求。

【范文评述】

本篇范文结构完整,内容丰富翔实,涵盖了试题表格中提供的所有细节,包括病人的个人信息、主要症状、家族史、生活习惯、过敏源等。本范文语言通顺,表述清晰,措辞符合医学英语用语规范,句式简单但信息全面。时态使用也妥帖无误,文中绝大部分句子为主动语态和一般现在时态,但根据具体情况,作者也采用了被动语态和现在完成时态表达了客观事实,展示了其良好的英语写作基础。从文中可以看出,本文作者有比较扎实的语法知识,所有的句子表达都没有语法错误。

医护英语水平考试（一级）

模拟训练（六）

听力文本

This is METS-1 listening test. There are four parts to the test, parts One, Two, Three, and Four. You will hear each part twice. Now, look at the instructions for Part One. You will hear five patients describing their pain. Decide where each patient has the pain. Write the appropriate letter A—H in each box. Mark the corresponding letter on your answer sheet. You will hear each conversation twice.

Here is an example:

Nurse (Woman): What's brought you here, Tim?
Patient (Man): My wrist has been throbbing since I fell in the street.

The answer is in the wrist, so write letter F in the box. Now we are ready to start.

Conversation 1

Nurse (Woman): Good afternoon, Mr. White. What brought you here?
Patient (Man): Well, I have had a pain in my stomach.

Conversation 2

Nurse (Woman): Good morning, Mr. Smith. What's the matter with you?
Patient (Man): Good morning. I have a sore throat.

Conversation 3

Nurse (Woman): Hello, Mr. Blaire. How are you feeling today?
Patient (Man): Not great. I still feel very tired and I still have a sore back.

Conversation 4

Nurse (Woman): How do you feel this morning, Louise?
Patient (Man): I feel terrible. I have a really bad headache and a stiff neck.

Conversation 5

Nurse (Woman): Good morning, Mr. Green. Can I help you?
Patient (Man): Well, I cut my hand at work and it looked like a bad cut.

This is the end of Part One. Now look at Part Two. You will hear a conversation of a nurse talking to a patient. For each of the following sentences, decide whether it is True (A) or False (B). Put a tick (√) in the relevant box. Mark the corresponding letter on your answer sheet. You will hear the conversation twice.

Nurse (Woman): Good afternoon, Mr. Gates. Tell me how you feel.
Patient (Man): Good afternoon, Mary. I have had a bad headache for almost a week. I can't sleep well because of the pain during night.
Nurse (Woman): Yes, I can see that from your looks. Did you take any kind of painkiller for your headache?
Patient (Man): No. I tried not to take any medicine for that, but it seems to be getting worse in the past two days.

Nurse (Woman): Can you show me exactly where you feel the headache, please?

Patient (Man): It's on the left side of my head. It comes and goes suddenly.

Nurse (Woman): How often does it occur?

Patient (Man): About every half an hour.

Nurse (Woman): OK. Do you have a family history of headache? Did anybody have a stroke or any other problem with the brain in your family in the past?

Patient (Man): No. I don't think so.

This is the end of Part Two. Now look at Part Three. You will hear a conversation between a patient and a chemist about taking medicine. For each of the following questions (or unfinished sentences), choose the correct answer A, B or C. Put a tick (√) in the relevant box. Mark the corresponding letter on your answer sheet. You will hear the conversation twice.

Chemist (Woman): Good morning, Mr. Brown. Can I help you?

Patient (Man): Um ... well, could you give me something for a cough? I feel I'm getting one.

Chemist (Woman): Is it a cough in the chest?

Patient (Man): No. It's a dry cough in my throat.

Chemist (Woman): Do you have any other symptoms?

Patient (Man): Well, I have a bit of a headache and I feel very tired.

Chemist (Woman): It sounds like you might be getting the flu. There's a flu going around at the moment. Lots of people have it. Here's the cough mixture for your throat and some painkillers for your headache.

Patient (Man): Er ... I can't read the dosage. How many do I take each time?

Chemist (Woman): You take one or two painkillers three or four times a day. But don't take more than eight within one day.

Patient (Man): OK. And the cough medicine?

Chemist (Woman): One or two spoonfuls every four hours.

Patient (Man): OK. Thank you very much.

Chemist (Woman): My pleasure.

This is the end of Part Three. Now look at Part Four. You will hear a conversation between a nurse and a patient. Fill in the blanks. Write the answers on your answer sheet. You will hear the conversation twice.

Nurse(Woman): Good morning. This is Dr. Johnson's office. What can I do for you?

Patient (Man): Yes, this is Paul Reed. I'd like to make an appointment to see Doctor Johnson for my teeth this week.

34

Nurse（Woman）：Well，let me have a look. I'm afraid he is fully booked on Monday and Tuesday.

Patient（Man）：How about Thursday?

Nurse（Woman）：Sorry，and I have to say he is also full on Thursday. So，will Wednesday be OK for you，Mr. Reed?

Patient（Man）：I have to work on Wednesday morning，but I will be free on Wednesday afternoon.

Nurse（Woman）：That's fine. Could I have your telephone number?

Patient（Man）：It's 83462269.

Nurse（Woman）：Well，what's your date of birth and do you have any health insurances?

Patient（Man）：I was born on the 3rd of January，1970. I have a health insurance and I'll take the health insurance card with me.

Nurse（Woman）：OK. See you on Wednesday afternoon，Mr. Reed.

This is the end of Part Four. You now have five minutes to write your answers on the answer sheet. You have one more minute. This is the end of the listening test.

参考答案及解析

Ⅰ Listening

Part One

1. E 本题中患者自述胃痛（in my stomach），故选 E。

2. H 本题中患者咽喉痛（a sore throat），故选 H。

3. C 本题中患者自述背疼（I still have a sore back），故选 C。

4. G 本题中患者头疼得厉害（a really bad headache），故选 G。

5. A 本题中患者手被割伤，且很严重，故选 A。

Part Two

6. B 患者头疼了一个星期，故本句错误。

7. A 患者晚上头疼得睡不着觉，故本句正确。

8. A 患者自述并没有针对头疼服用任何药，故本句正确。

9. A 患者描述头疼的部位在左侧，故本句正确。

10. B 患者陈述每半小时疼痛发作一次，故本句错误。

Part Three

11. B 患者觉得自己咳嗽（cough），故选 B。

12. C 患者描述其他症状有头疼（headache），故选 C。

13. C 针对咳嗽，药剂师建议服用止咳药（cough mixture），针对头疼药剂师建议服用止疼药（painkillers），故选 C。

14. B 药剂师建议止疼药一天不能超过八片（not more than eight），故选 B。

15. A 药剂师建议止咳药每四小时服用一次(every four hours),故选 A。

Part Four

16. Paul 根据患者回答来确定。

17. teeth 患者想看牙医。

18. 83462269 根据患者回答来确定。

19. January 患者出生于 1970 年 1 月 3 日。

20. Wednesday 患者最后定于周三下午看医生。

Ⅱ Reading and Writing

Part One

21. G 根据 vehicle 和 transport 判断,选 G。

22. E 根据 surgical operations 判断,选 E。

23. H 根据 a document of a patient's medical history 判断,选 H。

24. F 根据 cover the wounds 判断要用到敷料,故选 F。

25. D 根据 measures temperature 判断,选 D。

Part Two

26. C 根据 have your tooth checked 判断,选 C。

27. E 根据 get different kinds of medicine 判断,选 E。

28. A 题干中 put it in a high place 符合 A 中提到的 Keep Out Of Reach Of Children 的要求。

29. B 根据 measure your blood pressure at home 判断,选 B。

30. F 本题题干的 take one tablet half an hour before meals 属于用药指导,故选 F。

Part Three

31. D 上文是针对时间的提问,答案锁定在 D 和 G,又因是对结果的询问,所以回答 D。

32. A 上文患者问护士,术前他应该做些什么,故选 A。

33. E 患者提到他以前从来没有做过任何手术,故选 E。

34. F 护士安慰患者,放松点,医生和护士会帮助你的,故选 F。

35. G 患者问,他将什么时候接受手术,故选 G。

Part Four

36. A 定位第一段第一句"Diabetes is a chronic, metabolic disease characterized by elevated levels of blood sugar."

37. B 定位第一段第二行"leads over time to serious damage to the heart, blood vessels, eyes, kidneys, and nerves",没有提到 lungs。

38. A 定位第一段最后一句"Symptoms of high blood sugar include frequent urination, increased thirst, and increased hunger."

39. B 根据第二段第三行"The cause is unknown."判断选 B。

40. A 根据第二段第五行关于 type 2 diabetes 的介绍中提到的"It often results from overweight and not enough exercise."判断这属于二型糖尿病的诱因,故选 A。

41. A 定位第二段第四行"It is caused by the body's ineffective use of insulin."

42. A 定位第二段倒数第二句"In the past three decades the prevalence of type 2 diabetes has risen dramatically in countries of all income levels."

43. B 定位第二段最后一句"Gestational diabetes is the third main form and occurs when pregnant women without a previous history of diabetes develop high blood-sugar levels."

44. C 文中并未提到如何预防糖尿病。

45. A 定位最后一段最后一句"There is a globally agreed target to stop the rise in diabetes and obesity by 2025."

Part Five

46. A 这一句解释体重超重影响健康,根据搭配"so ... that"和句义选 A。

47. C 这一句是关于导致肥胖的原因,后面为介词 from,故选 C,构成搭配 result from。

48. E 肥胖产生原因有两个,吃得太多和动得太少,用 enough 修饰 exercise。

49. L 固定搭配 be high in。

50. I 前面是形容词 sedentary,所以后面要用名词,再根据上文及句义(现在人动得少),这属于一种静态的生活方式。

51. D 此处应该填副词,用来修饰动词 increased 且表示急剧增长,故选副词 rapidly。

52. F 从本空格前的形容词 increasing 来看,此空格应填名词,故选 F。

53. J 此句缺动词,且前面是 is,再结合句义,故选 affecting。

54. G 根据前面的 were 和后面的 in 判断,选 living。

55. B 固定搭配 be likely to。

Part Six

56.

Tips on Protecting Eyes

Eyes are very important to you, so you should be careful and know how to protect your eyes. As an adult, you should visit an eye doctor at least every two years to ensure good eye health. Eye drops are useful for treating and protecting your eyes. Watching a lot of TV and using mobile phone too much can cause eye strain and fatigue. What's more, you should always make sure to read in good lighting and take frequent breaks to rest your eyes. At last, it is also helpful for your eyes to eat nutrient-rich foods and get enough sleep.

【审题】

本题要求根据护眼建议,书写一篇不少于 80 个词的作文。在写作时,需要将这些建议用句子的形式完整地表达。注意:不可遗漏任何建议,标点符号要正确使用。时态的选择也是不可忽视的。这四个护眼建议是作文的主要内容,因此,本文时态应以一般现在时态为主。写作时,还要注意句子结构的完整性及句子之间的逻辑性,适当使用承转启合的连接词,并且文章的字数也应符合要求。

【范文评述】

本篇作文内容翔实，涵盖了试题中提供的所有要点，语言流畅，表述清晰。行文前，作者能仔细阅读"Tips on Protecting Eyes"中的每一个建议，并加以理解。文中的绝大部分句子为主动语态和一般现在时态，符合本文要求。从文中可以看出，本文作者有比较扎实的语法知识，能用不同的句型表达观点，并且所有的句子表达都没有语法错误。What's more …，At last 等结构和短语的运用使句与句之间的逻辑性更强，结构紧凑、完整。总之，本篇范文符合 METS 一级的写作要求，是一篇规范之作。

医护英语水平考试（一级）

模拟训练（七）

听力文本

This is METS-1 listening test. There are four parts to the test, parts One, Two, Three, and Four. You will hear each part twice. Now, look at the instructions for Part One. You will hear five patients describing their pain. Decide where each patient has the pain. Write the appropriate letter A—H in each box. Mark the corresponding letter on your answer sheet. You will hear each conversation twice.

Here is an example:

Nurse（Woman）：What brought you here, Tim?
Patient（Man）：My wrist has been throbbing since I fell in the street.

The answer is in the wrist, so write letter F in the box. Now we are ready to start.

Conversation 1

Nurse（Woman）：How do you feel this morning, Terry?
Patient（Man）：Awful. I've got a terrible headache.

Conversation 2

Nurse（Woman）：Are you all right, Joseph?
Patient（Man）：No. I've got a really bad stomachache. Possibly I have a fever.

Conversation 3

Nurse（Woman）：What brought you here, Clare?
Patient（Man）：My knee hurts a bit and I can't walk properly.

Conversation 4

Nurse（Man）：What happened to you, Tina?

Patient（Woman）：Just now I fell from bicycle and I have a sharp pain in my hands now.

Conversation 5

Nurse（Woman）：What's wrong with you, Sammy?

Patient（Man）：Yesterday I caught a cold and now I have a sore throat.

This is the end of Part One. Now look at Part Two. You will hear a conversation of a nurse talking to a patient. For each of the following sentences, decide whether it is True (A) or False (B). Put a tick (√) in the relevant box. Mark the corresponding letter on your answer sheet. You will hear the conversation twice.

Judy（Man）：Hello, Usha. How are feeling today?

Usha（Woman）：Hello, Judy. I feel a bit down today.

Judy（Man）：Oh, I'm sorry to hear that. Anything you want to tell me?

Usha（Woman）：Well ... um, I'm still in a lot of pain.

Judy（Man）：Oh, I see. You don't think the pain is getting any better with your treatment?

Usha（Woman）：No. I feel it's getting worse.

Judy（Man）：Mm, did you have radiotherapy yesterday?

Usha（Woman）：Yes, I had it yesterday morning. It made me feel quite sick.

Judy（Man）：Mm, I know. Radiotherapy can make you feel quite sick.

Usha（Woman）：And I don't feel like eating anything at all.

Judy（Man）：Why don't I get you some medicine for your pain and nausea?

Usha（Woman）：Good idea. Then I can have a rest.

Judy（Man）：I'll bring you the medicine right now.

Usha（Woman）：Thanks.

This is the end of Part Two. Now look at Part Three. You will hear a conversation between a nurse and a patient. For each of the following questions (or unfinished sentences), choose the correct answer A, B or C. Put a tick (√) in the relevant box. Mark the corresponding letter on your answer sheet. You will hear the conversation twice.

Angela（Woman）：Morning, Mr. Briggs. It's Angela. I'm here for your dressing. Can I come in?

Mr. Briggs（Man）：Hello, Angela. Come in, please.

Angela (Woman): Let me have a look at the wound to see how it's going.

Mr. Briggs (Man): OK. I'll put my leg up for you.

Angela (Woman): That's good. I'll take the bandage off first. Mm, well, it looks much better.

Mr. Briggs (Man): Ooh. But it still looks awful to me.

Angela (Woman): Actually, the skin around the wound is less red.

Mr. Briggs (Man): Yes. I suppose so.

Angela (Woman): The wound has got less pus in it.

Mr. Briggs (Man): That's good.

Angela (Woman): It doesn't have a bad odor now because the infection is better. And the wound is a bit smaller, too.

Mr. Briggs (Man): That's great.

Angela (Woman): Mr. Briggs, could I do the dressing now?

Mr. Briggs (Man): Thanks, Angela. Just wait a minute. I'd like to have a shower first.

This is the end of Part Three. Now look at Part Four. You will hear a conversation between two nurses. Fill in the blanks. Write the answers on your answer sheet. You will hear the conversation twice.

Helena (Woman): All right, Tom, let's get the next bag ready. Before we start, we need to wash our hands.

Tom (Man): Yes, of course.

Helena (Woman): First, we'll check the IV solution against the IV prescription.

Tom (Man): All right.

Helena (Woman): Next, I'm going to prime the line. Can you run the IV fluid through the IV tubing of the giving set?

Tom (Man): Yes, I can.

Helena (Woman): After we run this IV infusion through the IV infusion pump, we need to set the rate on the infusion pump.

Helena (Woman): Now we both have to sign the IV prescription.

Tom (Man): OK. Should we sign here?

Helena (Woman): That's right. The last thing is to write up the Fluid Balance Chart.

Tom (Man): OK. Where is the chart?

Helena (Woman): Here. Well done!

This is the end of Part Four. You now have five minutes to write your answers on the answer sheet. You have one more minute. This is the end of the listening test.

40

参考答案及解析

I Listening

Part One

1. H 本题中患者自述头疼(headache)，故选 H。

2. C 本题中患者自述胃疼(stomachache)，故选 C。

3. E 本题中患者自述膝盖疼(knee hurts)，故选 E。

4. A 本题中患者自述手疼(a sharp pain in my hands)，故选 A。

5. B 本题中患者自述喉咙疼(sore throat)，故选 B。

Part Two

6. B 根据对话内容，患者刚做完放疗，感觉恶心，吃不下东西，故本句错误。

7. A 患者觉得现在接受的治疗并没有缓解她的疼痛感，反而加剧了，故本句正确。

8. A 根据对话，患者现在正在接受放疗。故本句正确。

9. A 患者在对话中提到放疗让她感觉十分反胃，故本句正确。

10. A 对话最后，患者说需要好好休息一下，故本句正确。

Part Three

11. C 根据对话内容，护士给病人换敷料。首先，她将取下绷带，故选 C。

12. B 患者自述伤口十分恶心，故选 B。

13. B 护士说伤口周边的皮肤不怎么红了，故选 B。

14. C 护士说伤口范围正在逐渐缩小，故选 C。

15. B 对话最后，患者说想要先洗个澡，故选 B。

Part Four

16. hands 开篇时，女护士说开始进行输液前要先洗手。

17. solution 女护士说第一步为对照着静脉输液处方单核对药液。

18. line 女护士然后说，prime the line.

19. rate 输液开始前要先在输液泵上设置好滴速。

20. Chart 最后一步是在表单上做记录。

II Reading and Writing

Part One

21. G 用来注射的是注射器，故选 G。

22. D 用精油进行治疗的是芳香疗法，故选 D。

23. E 按摩身体某个部位缓解疼痛是按摩，故选 E。

24. C 口服或者通过注射来止痛的药物是止痛药，故选 C。

25. B 用针止痛是针灸疗法，故选 B。

Part Two

26. D 摇匀。

27. C 用水漱口。

28. A 避免日照。

29. B 避免含酒精饮料。

30. F 丢弃容器内所剩物。

Part Three

31. G 从上一句护士说"Do you have any trouble feeding yourself?",可以判断,这是一个一般疑问句,用 "Yes"或"No"来回答。故选 G。

32. D 从上一句护士说 "How could I help you?",患者的回答应该是 D。

33. B 上句护士说 OT 给你送来了一些工具帮助你用餐。下句患者应该是顺理成章地说 B。

34. E 护士说这是一个特殊的碗,患者的反应应该是 E。

35. C 护士下一句说这是一个防滑杯子,患者上一句应该说 "What about the cup in your left hand?",故选 C。

Part Four

36. B 文中第二段前两句 Mammograms can also be used to check for breast cancer after a lump or another sign or symptom of breast cancer has been found. This type of mammogram is called a diagnostic mammogram.

37. B 文中第三段第一句 Diagnostic mammograms take longer than screening mammograms because they involve more X-rays in order to obtain views of the breast from several angles.

38. A 文中第三段第一句 Diagnostic mammograms take longer than screening mammograms because they involve more X-rays in order to obtain views of the breast from several angles.

39. B 文中第四段最后一句 For example, some cancers cannot be found by a screening mammogram but may be found by a clinical breast exam.

40. B 文中最后一段最后一句 Breast self-exams alone have not been found to help reduce the number of deaths from breast cancer.

41. C 本题文中未提及。

42. B 最后一段第二句 Breast self-exams cannot replace regular screening mammograms or clinical breast exams.

43. C 本题文中未提及。

44. A 第三段最后一句 The technician may magnify an area to produce a detailed picture that can help the doctor make an accurate diagnosis.

45. A 第二段第三句 Signs of breast cancer may include pain, skin thickening, nipple discharge, or a change in breast size or shape.

Part Five

46. G 根据后面的 having a shower or going to the toilet,推断出应该是 daily activities。

47. H 本文的主题是如何处理让患者尴尬的事情,比如如厕,所以空缺处应该填写

embarrassing。

48. L 比如，尿失禁的患者可能会觉得十分羞愧而不去按护士铃呼叫护士。尿失禁 incontinent of urine。

49. B 呼叫铃 call bell 参考上题。

50. I It is important to do …

51. F 固定搭配 make sure。

52. D 尤其是老年患者 elderly patients。

53. K 假如老年患者尿失禁,轻视他们是不可取的。

54. J 总之,我们要给患者足够的时间处理他们的事情,不要不耐烦。

55. C 本文题目为 How to Manage Embarrassing Moments。

Part Six

56.

A Case Report

The patient Mr. James Boone was born on January 3,1982. He is a single, unmarried. He works as an engineer. His next of kin is his father,David Boone. His father's contact number is 01863 - 652984. He was admitted to hospital because of a car accident. He doesn't smoke cigarettes or drink alcohol. He has a family history of heart disease on his mother's side. And he is allergic to shellfish,one kind of the seafood.

【审题】

本题考查考生以病例表为基本信息,要求考生写一篇不少于80词的作文。其内容应包括:患者姓名、出生年月、职业、婚姻状况、直系亲属及其联系方式、入院原因以及过敏史等等。本题中患者病例表所提供的信息比较齐全,所以只需将表中的单词或词组用适当的形式连成句子即可。写作中要注意信息的处理,不可遗漏任何重要信息,必要时可以重新组合,并使用适当的连词使前后句子语意连贯,重点突出。可参考的重点词汇、句型为 be admitted to hospital,because of,be allergic to,have a disease on … side 等。

【范文评述】

本篇范文内容翔实,涵盖了试题中提供的所有细节,包括患者的姓名、职业、出生年月、婚姻状况、入院原因、家族史、过敏史等。文章语言通顺,结构完整,无病句或其他语法错误。在时态的使用方面也十分妥帖,如在介绍患者基本情况主要用一般现在时,因陈述既定事实,如入院原因,使用一般过去时,因其内容为已经发生过的事情。在语言使用上也有可圈可点之处,如第五句使用 because of 的原因状语从句。总体来说,这篇范文结构完整,用语规范,无语法错误。